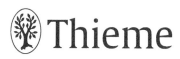

RadCases Plus Q&A Pediatric Imaging
Second Edition

Authored by

Richard B. Gunderman, MD, PhD, MPH
The John A. Campbell Professor of Radiology
Chancellor's Professor of Radiology, Pediatrics,
   Medical Education, Philosophy, Liberal Arts,
   Philanthropy, and Medical Humanities and
   Health Studies
Indiana University
Indianapolis, Indiana

Lisa R. Delaney, MD
Assistant Professor
Department of Radiology
Indiana University School of Medicine
Indianapolis, Indiana

Series Editors

Jonathan M. Lorenz, MD, FSIR
Professor of Radiology
Section of Interventional Radiology
The University of Chicago
Chicago, Illinois

Hector Ferral, MD
Senior Medical Educator
NorthShore University HealthSystem
Evanston, Illinois

370 illustrations

Thieme
New York • Stuttgart • Delhi • Rio de Janeiro

Executive Editor: William Lamsback
Managing Editors: J. Owen Zurhellen IV & Kenneth Schubach
Editorial Assistant: Holly Bullis
Director, Editorial Services: Mary Jo Casey
Production Editor: Teresa Exley, Absolute Service, Inc.
International Production Director: Andreas Schabert
Editorial Director: Sue Hodgson
International Marketing Director: Fiona Henderson
International Sales Director: Louisa Turrell
Director of Institutional Sales: Adam Bernacki
Senior Vice President and Chief Operating Officer: Sarah Vanderbilt
President: Brian D. Scanlan
Printer: King Printing

Library of Congress Cataloging-in-Publication Data

Names: Gunderman, Richard B., editor. | Delaney, Lisa R., editor.
Title: RadCases plus Q&A pediatric imaging / edited by
    Richard B. Gunderman, Lisa R. Delaney.
Other titles: Pediatric imaging (Gunderman) | RadCases plus Q and A
    pediatric imaging
Description: Second edition. | New York : Thieme, [2019] | Series:
    RadCases | Preceded by Pediatric imaging / edited by
    Richard B. Gunderman, Lisa R. Delaney. 2010. | Includes
    bibliographical references and index. |
    Identifiers: LCCN 2018038407 (print) | LCCN 2018038630
    (ebook) | ISBN 9781626235205 | ISBN 9781626235199 |
    ISBN 9781626235205 (e-ISBN)
Subjects: | MESH: Diagnostic Imaging | Child | Infant | Case Reports
Classification: LCC RJ51.D5 (ebook) | LCC RJ51.D5 (print) | NLM
    WN 240 | DDC 618.92/00754—dc23
LC record available at https://lccn.loc.gov/2018038407

Important note: Medicine is an ever-changing science undergoing continual development. Research and clinical experience are continually expanding our knowledge, in particular our knowledge of proper treatment and drug therapy. Insofar as this book mentions any dosage or application, readers may rest assured that the authors, editors, and publishers have made every effort to ensure that such references are in accordance with **the state of knowledge at the time of production of the book.**

Nevertheless, this does not involve, imply, or express any guarantee or responsibility on the part of the publishers in respect to any dosage instructions and forms of applications stated in the book. **Every user is requested to examine carefully** the manufacturers' leaflets accompanying each drug and to check, if necessary in consultation with a physician or specialist, whether the dosage schedules mentioned therein or the contraindications stated by the manufacturers differ from the statements made in the present book. Such examination is particularly important with drugs that are either rarely used or have been newly released on the market. Every dosage schedule or every form of application used is entirely at the user's own risk and responsibility. The authors and publishers request every user to report to the publishers any discrepancies or inaccuracies noticed. If errors in this work are found after publication, errata will be posted at www.thieme.com on the product description page.

Some of the product names, patents, and registered designs referred to in this book are in fact registered trademarks or proprietary names even though specific reference to this fact is not always made in the text. Therefore, the appearance of a name without designation as proprietary is not to be construed as a representation by the publisher that it is in the public domain.

Copyright © 2019 by Thieme Medical Publishers, Inc.
Thieme Publishers New York
333 Seventh Avenue, New York, NY 10001 USA
+1 800 782 3488, customerservice@thieme.com

Thieme Publishers Stuttgart
Rüdigerstrasse 14, 70469 Stuttgart, Germany
+49 [0]711 8931 421, customerservice@thieme.de

Thieme Publishers Delhi
A-12, Second Floor, Sector-2, Noida-201301
Uttar Pradesh, India
+91 120 45 566 00, customerservice@thieme.in

Thieme Publishers Rio de Janeiro, Thieme Publicações Ltda.
Edifício Rodolpho de Paoli, 25° andar
Av. Nilo Peçanha, 50 – Sala 2508
Rio de Janeiro 20020-906 Brasil
+55 21 3172-2297/+55 21 3172-1896
www.thiemerevinter.com.br

Cover design: Thieme Publishing Group
Typesetting by Absolute Service, Inc.
Printed in the United States by King Printing

5 4 3 2 1

ISBN 978-1-62623-519-9

Also available as an e-book:
eISBN 978-1-62623-520-5

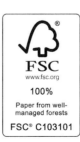

FSC
www.fsc.org
100%
Paper from well-managed forests
FSC® C103101

Dedicated to Laura, Rebecca, Peter, David, and John.

– RBG

Dedicated to Jill Voltmer and Ashley Carman, whose selflessness forever changed our lives and can never be repaid. We will never take for granted what you did for us.

– LRD

Series Preface

As enthusiastic partners in radiology education, we continue our mission to ease the exhaustion and frustration shared by residents and the families of residents engaged in radiology training! In launching the second edition of the RadCases series, our intent is to expand rather than replace this already rich study experience that has been tried, tested, and popularized by residents around the world. In each subspecialty edition, we serve up 100 new, carefully chosen cases to raise the bar in our effort to assist residents in tackling the daunting task of assimilating massive amounts of information. RadCases second edition primes and expands on concepts found in the first edition with important variations on prior cases, updated diagnostic and management strategies, and new pathologic entities. Our continuing goal is to combine the popularity and portability of printed books with the adaptability, exceptional quality, and interactive features of an electronic case-based format. The new cases will be added to the existing electronic database to enrich the interactive environment of high-quality images that allows residents to arrange study sessions, quickly extract and master information, and prepare for theme-based radiology conferences.

We owe a debt of gratitude to our own residents and to the many radiology trainees who have helped us create, adapt, and improve the format and content of RadCases by weighing in with suggestions for new cases, functions, and formatting. Back by popular demand is the concise, point-by-point presentation of the Essential Facts of each case in an easy-to-read, bulleted format, and a short, critical differential starting with the actual diagnosis. This approach is easy on exhausted eyes and encourages repeated priming of important information during quick reviews, a process we believe is critical to radiology education. New since the prior edition is the addition of a question-and-answer section for each case to reinforce key concepts.

The intent of the printed books is to encourage repeated priming in the use of critical information by providing a portable group of exceptional core cases to master. Unlike the authors of other case-based radiology review books, we removed the guesswork by providing clear annotations and descriptions for all images. In our opinion, there is nothing worse than being unable to locate a subtle finding on a poorly reproduced image even after one knows the final diagnosis.

The electronic cases expand on the printed book and provide a comprehensive review of the entire specialty. Thousands of cases are strategically designed to increase the resident's knowledge by providing exposure to a spectrum of case examples—from basic to advanced—and by exploring "Aunt Minnies," unusual diagnoses, and variability within a single diagnosis. The search engine allows the resident to create individualized daily study lists that are not limited by factors such as radiology subsection. For example, tailor today's study list to cases involving tuberculosis and include cases in every subspecialty and every system of the body. Or study only thoracic cases, including those with links to cardiology, nuclear medicine, and pediatrics. Or study only musculoskeletal cases. The choice is yours.

As enthusiastic partners in this project, we started small and, with the encouragement, talent, and guidance of Timothy Hiscock and William Lamsback at Thieme Publishers, we have further raised the bar in our effort to assist residents in tackling the daunting task of assimilating massive amounts of information. We are passionate about continuing this journey and will continue to expand the series, adapt cases based on direct feedback from residents, and increase the features intended for board review and self-assessment. First and foremost, we thank our medical students, residents, and fellows for allowing us the privilege to participate in their educational journey.

Jonathan M. Lorenz, MD, FSIR
Hector Ferral, MD

Preface

It is an immense privilege to practice pediatric radiology. Compared to other medical specialists, the radiologist is privileged to peer inside the living human body and contribute to the diagnosis and care of an unusually large number of patients. Compared to other radiologists, pediatric specialists have the opportunity to evaluate all organ systems with every major imaging modality. Nowhere else in radiology is the growth and development of the patient so crucial to care. Above all, pediatric radiology provides an opportunity to contribute to the care of perhaps the most vulnerable and precious patients of all, at all stages from prenatal life through adolescence. It is a blessing to be able to count ourselves among a long line of esteemed colleagues, whose shoulders have provided a perch from which all who study pediatric radiology can see far.

Richard B. Gunderman, MD, PhD
Lisa R. Delaney, MD

Acknowledgments

Many people have contributed to this work: our colleagues in pediatric radiology at Indiana University, from whom we have learned so much and with whom it remains a privilege to work side by side each day, including Brandon Brown, Matthew Cooper, Donald Corea, Francis Marshalleck, Boaz Karmazyn, Megan Marine, and Matthew Wanner, as well as our recently retired colleague, Mervyn Cohen. Lisa Ferguson and Carlene Webb-Burton provided superb administrative support. RBG also thanks Kelsey Hilaire, Luke Flood, and especially Nathan Gruenhagen for help in preparing many of the cases. Above all, our deepest thanks go to our families for their great patience and support as we labored over this project.

Case 1

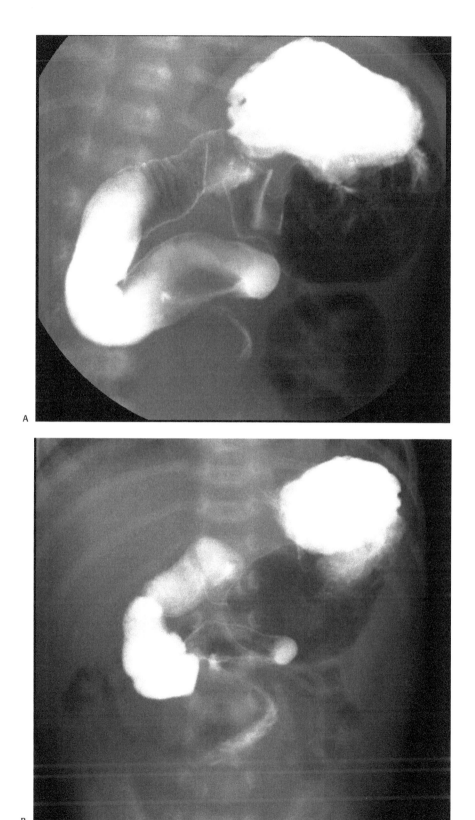

A

B

A 27-day-old boy presents with vomiting that turned bilious on day 2.

■ Imaging Findings

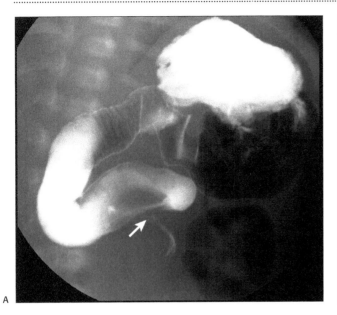 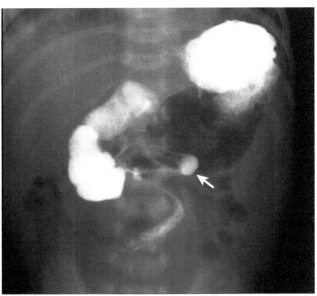

(A) Oblique view from a barium upper gastrointestinal (GI) examination demonstrates dilation of the proximal duodenum that tapers to a beaklike appearance, followed distally by a helical or corkscrew configuration of the distal duodenum (*arrow*). **(B)** Frontal view from the same barium upper GI examination demonstrates a corkscrew appearance of the distal duodenum. The duodenal–jejunal junction (*arrow*) is positioned too caudal to the duodenal bulb.

■ Differential Diagnosis

- **Midgut volvulus:** The key imaging findings of midgut volvulus include an abnormal position of the duodenal–jejunal junction, in which radiographic contrast does not cross completely over to the left side of the spine, and a corkscrew configuration of the distal duodenum.
- *Gastroenteritis:* Most infants who present with bilious vomiting do not have an anatomic abnormality and instead are suffering from a functional condition such as gastroenteritis or feeding intolerance.
- *Congenital duodenal obstruction:* Conditions such as duodenal atresia and duodenal webs can be associated with bilious vomiting when the point of obstruction is distal to the ampulla of Vater.

■ Essential Facts

- Midgut volvulus occurs in patients with intestinal malrotation, whose small bowel mesentery has an abnormally short mesenteric root and is therefore prone to twisting or volvulus.
- Midgut volvulus involves twisting of the bowel around the axis of the superior mesenteric artery, which can cause ischemia and infarction of the bowel.
- Many patients with malrotation also have Ladd bands, abnormal adhesion-like fibrous bands that can cause intestinal obstruction independent of volvulus.
- Surgical correction via the Ladd procedure involves untwisting the bowel and fixing it to the peritoneal wall to prevent future volvulus, as well as lysis of Ladd bands.

■ Other Imaging Findings

- Plain radiographs may be normal, particularly if the stomach and proximal duodenum have been decompressed by vomiting or passage of a nasogastric tube.
- Cross-sectional imaging such as abdominal ultrasound or CT may show an abnormal relationship of the superior mesenteric artery and vein, with the vein lying to the left of the artery.
- Cross-sectional imaging may also show a helical or swirling of bowel around the axis of the superior mesenteric artery, best appreciated when scrolling through axial images.

✓ Pearls and ✗ Pitfalls

- ✓ In cases where the position of the duodenal–jejunal junction is equivocal, the progression of radiographic contrast can be followed through to the cecum, which is in its normal position in the right lower quadrant in only 20% of patients with malrotation.
- ✗ Note that patients who have undergone the Ladd procedure will still have malrotated bowel, with the small bowel on the right and large bowel on the left.

Case 2

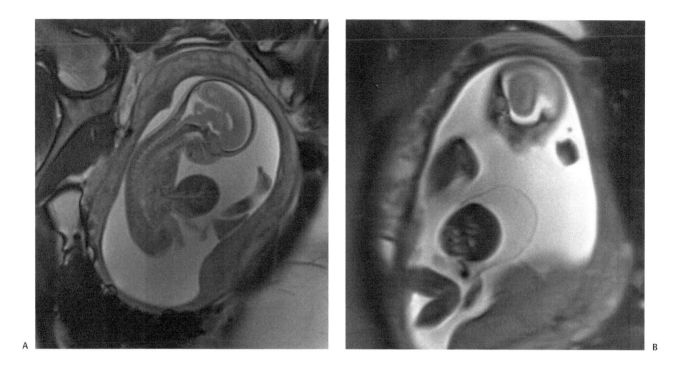

A   B

▨ Clinical Presentation

A fetus at 21 weeks' gestational age with abdominal wall defect seen on fetal ultrasound image.

▪ Imaging Findings

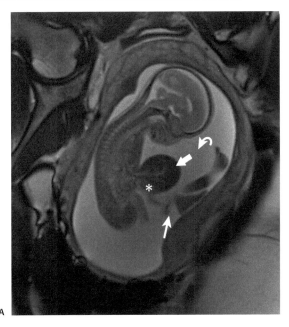
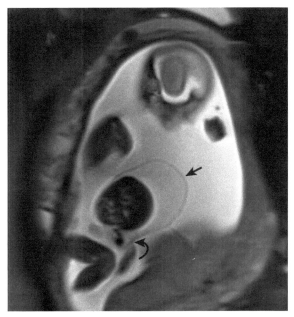

(A) Sagittal true fast imaging with steady-state precession (TrueFISP) fetal MR image. Part of the liver (*thick arrow*) and a small amount of bowel (*asterisk*) are seen outside of the abdominal cavity. There is a curvilinear membrane (*curved arrow*) covering the defect. The umbilical cord (*arrow*) inserts on the inferior aspect of the membrane. **(B)** Sagittal T2 half-Fourier acquisition single-shot turbo spin-echo (HASTE) fetal MR image. The hernia sac (*arrow*) is better delineated on this image. The umbilical cord insertion onto the sac (*curved arrow*) again can be seen.

▪ Differential Diagnosis

- **Fetal omphalocele:** A congenital midline abdominal wall defect with abdominal contents herniating into a sac onto which the umbilical cord inserts is consistent with an omphalocele.
- *Gastroschisis:* These abdominal wall defects are usually to the right of midline and are not covered by a membrane. The umbilical cord inserts normally on the abdominal wall, not on the defect.
- *Physiologic gut herniation:* Loops of bowel should never be seen outside of the abdominal cavity beyond 13 weeks of gestational age. In addition, physiologic herniation should only contain bowel loops, not liver.

▪ Essential Facts

- Associated anomalies are frequent and include cardiac, genitourinary, skeletal, and central nervous system. In addition, omphaloceles are associated with multiple syndromes including trisomies, Turner syndrome, Klinefelter syndrome, and others.
- Detection of associated anomalies is crucial for prognosis. The mortality rate is very high with any associated defect and severely high with associated chromosomal or cardiovascular anomalies. An isolated omphalocele has a much better prognosis.

▪ Other Imaging Findings

- Almost always initially discovered on fetal ultrasound image demonstrating multiple bowel loops herniating into a membrane-covered defect.
- Umbilical cord insertion is always on the membrane covering the herniation.
- Allantoic cyst in the umbilical cord is common.

✓ Pearls and ✗ Pitfalls

- ✓ Associated anomalies appear to be more frequent the earlier the omphalocele occurs in gestation and in smaller omphaloceles that contain only bowel.
- ✗ If the omphalocele ruptures, the membrane covering the herniated contents will be difficult to visualize and can be difficult to distinguish from gastroschisis.

Case 3

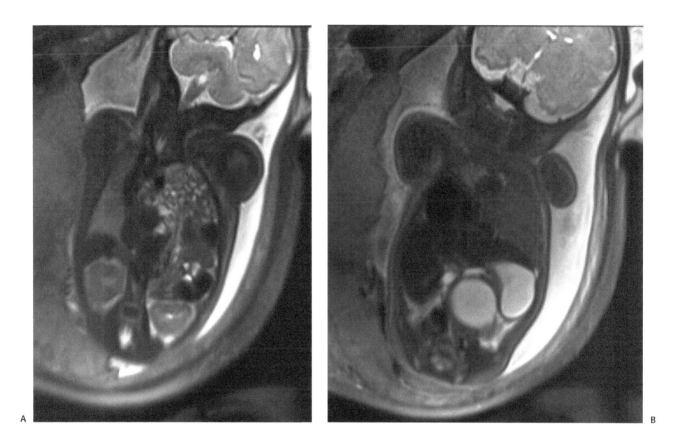

A   B

▓ Clinical Presentation

A fetus at 38 weeks' gestational age with concern for chest mass on fetal ultrasound image.

■ Imaging Findings

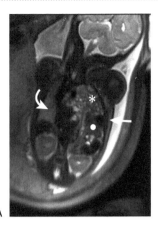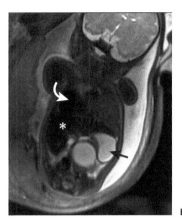

(A) Coronal half-Fourier acquisition single-shot turbo spin-echo (HASTE) fetal MR image. There are multiple loops of small bowel (*asterisk*), colon (*arrow*), and spleen (*dot*) in the left chest cavity causing mass effect on the normal right lung (*curved arrow*). **(B)** Coronal HASTE fetal MR image. The liver (*asterisk*) and stomach (*arrow*) are not herniated into the chest cavity. The heart (*curved arrow*) is displaced to the right.

■ Differential Diagnosis

- ***Congenital diaphragmatic hernia (CDH):*** Abdominal contents in the hemithorax is consistent with CDH.
- *Congenital pulmonary airway malformations (CPAM):* Although this also appears as fluid-filled cysts in the hemithorax, the cysts are not typically tubular like bowel and they are more uniform in appearance than a CDH that contains bowel and organs.
- *Bronchopulmonary sequestration (BPS):* These are typically well-defined and triangular in shape and homogeneously high T2 signal. Often, a feeding vessel from the aorta can be identified.

■ Essential Facts

- CDH can occur on either the left or right side. It is rarely bilateral.
- When CDH occurs on the right, liver is always herniated along with variable amounts of bowel and stomach.
- Associated anomalies include BPS, cardiac anomalies, aneuploidy, and multiple syndromes.

■ Other Imaging Findings

- Fetal MRI can be used to calculate a lung to head ratio and to measure fetal lung volumes, both of which help to predict outcomes based on lung hypoplasia.

- The cardiomediastinum shifts away from the hernia.
- Bowel loops are absent in the abdomen.
- On fetal ultrasonography, a CDH often appears as a cystic lung mass. In addition, if the stomach and small bowel are at the same transverse level as the heart on the four-chamber view on fetal ultrasound image, this confirms CDH.
- On fetal ultrasound image of a right CDH, color Doppler imaging may demonstrate leftward bowing of the umbilical segment of the portal vein, and portal branches to the lateral segment of the left lobe may course toward or above the diaphragm.

✓ Pearls and ✗ Pitfalls

- ✓ Most common on the left side.
- ✓ The degree of pulmonary hypoplasia, mediastinal shift, early diagnosis, and location of the liver (above or below the hemidiaphragm) all affect prognosis.
- ✓ MRI can reliably distinguish CPAM, BPS, and CDH, which is crucial for perinatal planning.
- ✗ No single parameter has been found to strongly correlate with survival or need for extracorporeal membrane oxygenation; however, there is a composite prognostic index used at some centers that may more strongly correlate with outcomes.

Case 4

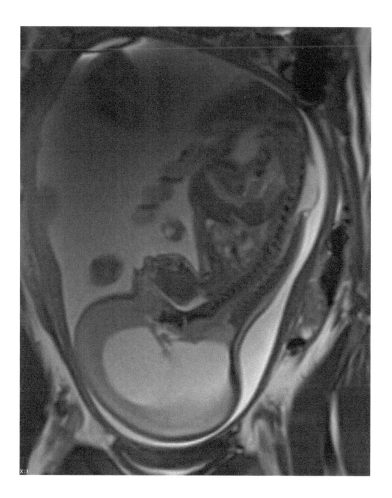

A fetus at 28 weeks' gestational age with hydrocephalus on fetal ultrasound image.

■ Imaging Findings

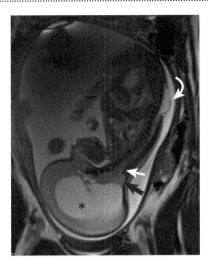

(A) Sagittal true fast imaging with steady-state precession (TrueFISP) fetal MR image. Marked hydrocephalus (*asterisk*) is seen with a small posterior fossa (*black arrow*). There is herniation of the cerebellar tonsils to the level of the cervical spine (*white arrow*). From approximately T12 to L4, there is absence of the posterior elements and a myelomeningocele sac (*curved arrow*).

■ Differential Diagnosis

- **Chiari III malformation:** A small posterior fossa with descent of the brainstem and cerebellum as well as a myelomeningocele is characteristic of Chiari II malformation.
- *Chiari I malformation:* This does have caudal descent of the cerebellar tonsils but would not have the associated myelomeningocele. These are often asymptomatic until adulthood.
- *Chiari II malformation:* This has features of Chiari II, but instead of a lumbar myelomeningocele, there is an occipital or high cervical encephalocele.

■ Essential Facts

- Myelomeningocele is defined as the protrusion of neural elements and meninges through a bony spinal defect. It is the most common form of neural tube defect.
- Chiari II malformation is also known as Arnold–Chiari malformation.
- Causes varying degrees of paralysis, bladder and bowel morbidity, and developmental delay.
- Studies have shown that the higher the level and larger the size of the myelomeningocele as well as an absence in membranous covering are associated with increasingly adverse outcomes.
- Early causes of mortality include brainstem dysfunction, ventriculitis, and shunt-related complications. Renal disease is the main cause of mortality later in life.

■ Other Imaging Findings

- Other findings of Chiari II in the brain can include colpocephaly, inferior pointing of the lateral ventricles, fenestration of the falx cerebri with interdigitation of the gyri across midline, enlargement of the massa intermedia, tectal beaking, and subependymal gray matter heterotopia.
- In the axial plane of the spine, the open spinal dysraphism is identified as absence of the overlying muscle and skin.
- Can be associated with club foot, scoliosis, and Lückenschädel skull.

✓ Pearls and ✗ Pitfalls

- ✓ When there is a myelomeningocele, there is almost always a small posterior fossa and associated findings, and vice versa.
- ✓ On prenatal ultrasound image, the lemon sign (concavity of the frontal bones) and the banana cerebellar sign (cerebellum tightly wrapped around the brainstem) can be seen.
- ✗ The lemon sign on prenatal ultrasound image usually is not seen past 24 weeks' gestational age.
- ✗ Myelomeningoceles are associated with Chiari II malformations, but meningoceles are not.

Case 5

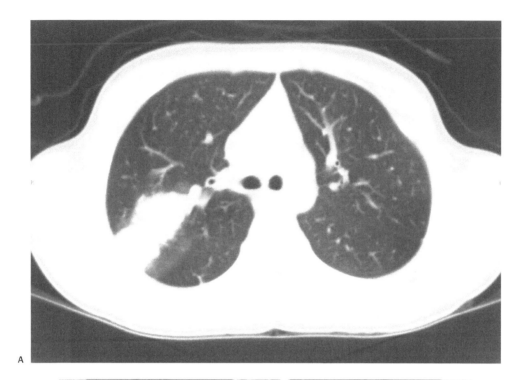

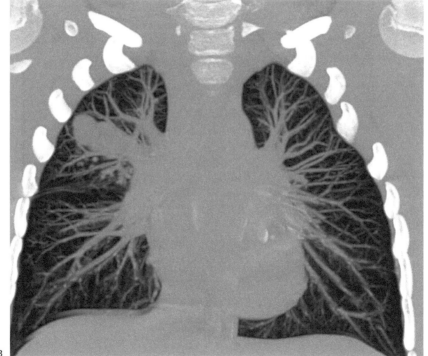

■ Clinical Presentation

A 10-year-old boy with cystic fibrosis exacerbation.

■ Imaging Findings

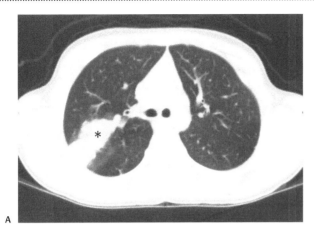
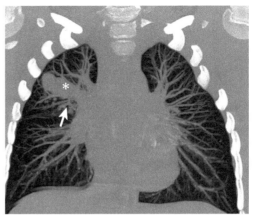

(A) Axial CT image of the chest. There is a tubular soft tissue density extending from the right hilum to the pleura (*asterisk*). **(B)** Coronal maximum intensity projection image of the chest. Seen again is the tubular opacity extending from the hilum in the right upper lobe (*asterisk*). In addition, along the inferior edge of the tubular density, there is tree-in-bud density (*arrow*).

■ Differential Diagnosis

- ***Allergic bronchopulmonary aspergillosis (ABPA):*** Saccular bronchiectasis filled with soft tissue density is consistent with a bronchocele. This combined with the history of cystic fibrosis should raise concern of ABPA.
- *Bronchial atresia:* Bronchoceles are also seen in bronchial atresia. They are usually surrounded by an area of hyperinflation and decreased vascular markings. In addition, this is not associated with cystic fibrosis.
- *Endobronchial lesion/foreign body:* Again, this could be associated with air-trapping but is not associated with cystic fibrosis.

■ Essential Facts

- ABPA is a hypersensitivity reaction to *Aspergillus* that occurs in patients with cystic fibrosis or asthma.
- *Aspergillus* grows in the airway, leading to bronchospasm and bronchial wall edema and causing bronchial wall damage and bronchiectasis.
- Segmental and subsegmental bronchi become filled with mucus, *Aspergillus*, and eosinophils.

■ Other Imaging Findings

- On chest X-ray, findings of asthma or cystic fibrosis may be present with superimposed fleeting opacities representing eosinophilic pneumonia.
- Mucoid impaction in dilated bronchi may appear masslike or branching and may cause atelectasis.
- CT findings include fleeting opacities, bronchiectasis, and bronchoceles (mucus-filled dilated bronchi). Findings are predominantly upper lobe in distribution.
- Bronchoceles can be described as finger-in-glove; tram-line shadows; bandlike (toothpaste) shadows; and sometimes "V," inverted "V," or "Y" shaped.
- If left untreated, ABPA can lead to extensive bronchiectasis and fibrosis.

✓ Pearls and ✗ Pitfalls

✓ In ~30% of patients, the mucus becomes calcified and has high density on CT images (the mucus plug is visually denser than the paraspinal muscles).

✓ Many patients cough up thick mucus plugs that may be orange in color.

✗ *Aspergillus* can cause many different findings in the lungs depending on the patient's comorbidities and amount of fungus present.

Case 6

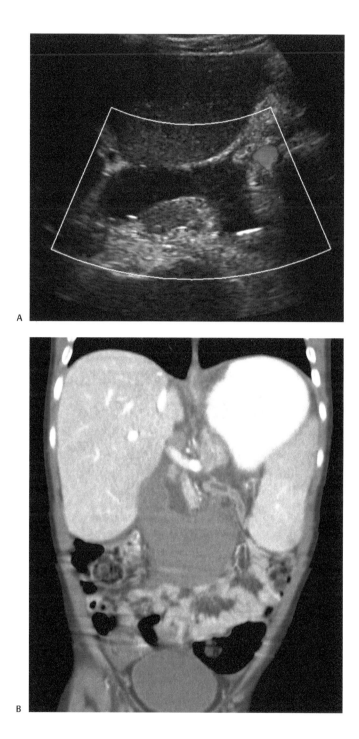

■ Clinical Presentation

An 8-year-old with abdominal pain after a fall.

◼ Imaging Findings

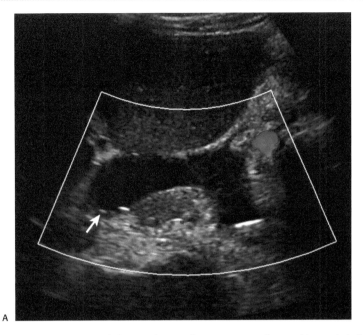
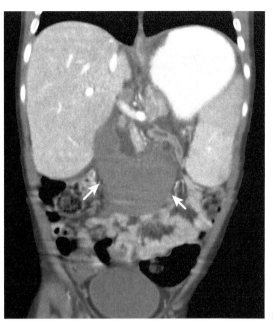

(A) Transverse abdominal ultrasound image demonstrates an elongated hypoechoic fluid collection behind the left lobe of the liver (*arrow*). **(B)** Coronal postcontrast CT scan demonstrates a hypodense fluid collection in the expected location of the distal duodenum (*arrows*).

◼ Differential Diagnosis

- **Duodenal hematoma:** The shape of the fluid collection follows the course of the distal duodenum, and its slight hyperintensity compared to the small amount of adjacent ascites suggests a hematoma.
- *Pancreatic pseudocyst:* Pancreatic pseudocysts in the lesser sac can assume an elongated shape, but it would be unusual for one to parallel the course of the distal duodenum so closely.
- *Duodenal duplication cyst:* Such cysts are typically found along the wall of the duodenum, but they do not typically have such an elongated shape and their walls should demonstrate the "bowel signature," which is not seen here.

◼ Essential Facts

- Associated with lap belt ecchymosis, handlebar injury, and child abuse.
- Patients commonly present with abdominal pain and vomiting.
- Most duodenal hematomas resolve spontaneously without surgery.

◼ Other Imaging Findings

- Traumatic duodenal hematomas are often associated with other injuries involving such structures as the pancreas and liver.
- Large hematomas such as this can be associated with duodenal obstruction.
- Over days, the density and echogenicity of a duodenal hematoma will tend to decrease.

✓ Pearls and ✗ Pitfalls

- ✓ In some cases of duodenal obstruction, it may be necessary to place a nasojejunal tube to permit feeding.
- ✗ It is important not to overlook findings of duodenal perforation, such as extraluminal gas, extravasated contrast, and discontinuities in the duodenal wall.

Case 7

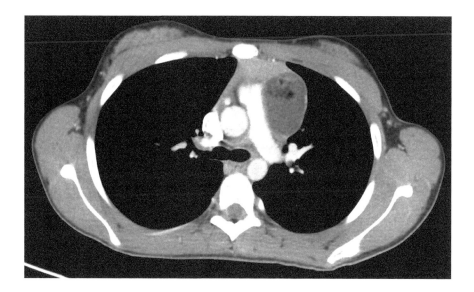

■ Clinical Presentation

A 13-year-old girl with a chest mass.

■ Imaging Findings

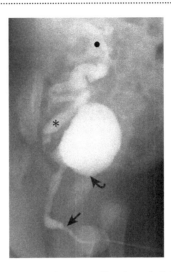

(A) Oblique view from a voiding cystourethrogram. There is an abrupt change in caliber (*arrow*) of the penile urethra with upstream dilation. There is mild trabeculation of the bladder wall (*curved arrow*) with right vesicoureteral reflux to the dilated, tortuous ureter (*asterisk*) and distended right renal collecting system (*dot*).

■ Differential Diagnosis

- **Anterior urethral valve (AUV):** The abrupt change in caliber of the penile urethra is consistent with AUV. Furthermore, the trabeculation of the bladder and severe vesicoureteral reflux are due to the significant lower urinary tract obstruction.
- *Posterior urethral valve (PUV):* The urethral dilation in PUVs is in the posterior (prostatic) urethra.
- *Prune belly (Eagle–Barrett) syndrome:* Prune belly syndrome shares some similarities of AUVs including a dilated urethra, trabeculation of the bladder, tortuosity of the ureters, and vesicoureteral reflux. Other important findings in prune belly include bulging flanks due to absence of the abdominal wall musculature and cryptorchidism. Other genitourinary findings of prune belly can include scaphoid urethra, urachal diverticulum, and opacification of the utricle.

■ Essential Facts

- AUVs may be found anywhere in the anterior urethra.
- PUVs are 15 to 30 times more common than AUVs.

■ Other Imaging Findings

- The valve itself may appear as a linear filling defect along the ventral wall.
- Alternatively, the valve itself may not be seen and is only indicated by a dilated urethra ending in a smooth bulge or an abrupt change in the caliber of the dilated urethra.
- Vesicoureteral reflux occurs in one third of cases.
- A trabeculated bladder with diverticula and a urethral diverticulum may also be seen.
- AUVs may be associated with urethral diverticula. Some consider them as separate entities, whereas others consider them part of the same entity.

✓ Pearls and ✕ Pitfalls

✓ Valves of Guerin are AUVs occurring in the most distal aspect of the urethra, the fossa navicularis.
✕ Patients with AUV have extremely variable presentations depending upon the degree of obstruction and the patient's age. Symptoms can range from urinary incontinence and retention with a weak urinary stream to infection, urosepsis, and renal failure.

Case 9

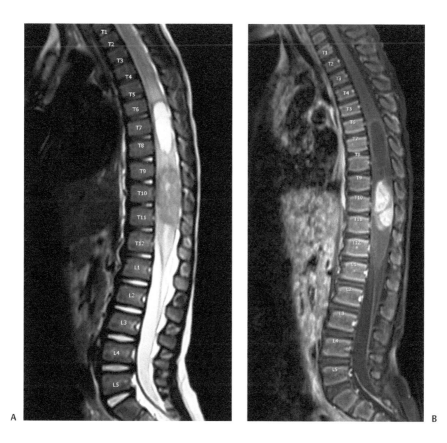

A

B

■ Clinical Presentation

A 4-year-old boy with unsteady gait.

■ Imaging Findings

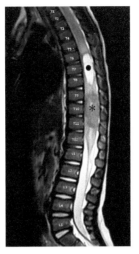
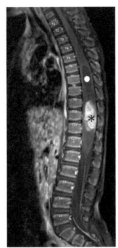

(A) Sagittal T2-weighted MR image of the spine. There is a large, ovoid, expansile intramedullary mass (*asterisk*) within the lower thoracic spinal cord from approximately T9 to T11. It has predominately low T2 signal but has some central increased T2 signal. Superior to this mass from approximately T6 to T8, there is an expansile cystic lesion (*dot*) with a rim of low T2 signal. **(B)** Sagittal T1 fat-saturated postcontrast image of the spine. There is contrast enhancement of the solid mass (*asterisk*) from T9 to T11 but not of the cystic mass (*dot*).

■ Differential Diagnosis

- **Spinal cord astrocytoma:** An enhancing, infiltrating mass that expands the spinal cord is consistent with an astrocytoma.
- *Spinal cord ependymoma:* These are uncommon in children but can appear similar to astrocytomas of the spinal cord. Ependymomas more often contain hemorrhage and are usually more well-defined than astrocytomas.
- *Syringohydromyelia:* This is a nonenhancing cystlike cavity in the spinal cord that is usually associated with a malformation such as Chiari I, spinal dysraphism, Dandy–Walker, or diastematomyelia.

■ Essential Facts

- Astrocytoma is the most common spinal cord neoplasm in children.
- Subarachnoid dissemination may occur.

■ Other Imaging Findings

- Mild scoliosis, widened intrapedicular distance, and bone erosion may be seen on plain film.
- On CT image, cord expansion can often be identified. The tumor itself may be difficult to resolve; however, it will usually enhance.
- Intratumoral and peritumoral cysts and surrounding edema are common.
- Astrocytomas may appear largely extramedullary.
- Involvement of the entire spinal cord (holocord involvement) is common in children.

✓ Pearls and ✕ Pitfalls

- ✓ Astrocytomas arise in the cord parenchyma, whereas ependymomas arise in the central canal.
- ✕ In one series, 20 to 30% of astrocytomas did not enhance.

Case 10

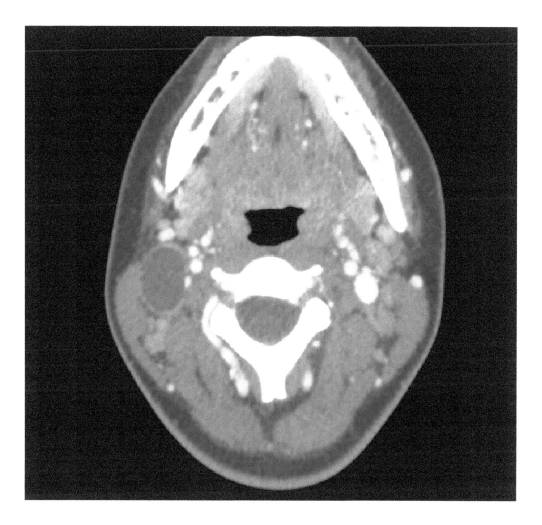

■ Clinical Presentation

A 15-year-old girl with a lump in her neck.

■ Imaging Findings

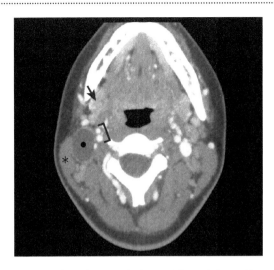

(A) Axial postcontrast CT image of the neck. Just deep to the right sternocleidomastoid muscle (*asterisk*), posterolateral to the right submandibular gland (*arrow*), and lateral to the right internal carotid artery and jugular vein (*bracket*) is a well-circumscribed fluid density lesion (*dot*) with a smooth, thin rim of peripheral enhancement.

■ Differential Diagnosis

- **Second branchial cleft cyst (type II):** This is the classic location of a branchial cleft cyst.
- *Thyroglossal duct cyst:* Typically, these are midline or slightly off midline.
- *Suppurative lymph node:* Although a suppurative lymph node could be low density with a thin rim of enhancement, this is fairly large for a lymph node and there are no other reactive lymph nodes in the area.

■ Essential Facts

- There are four types of second branchial cleft cysts, classified by location. Type II is the most common.
- Branchial cleft cysts usually present as a painless, fluctuant masses in the lateral neck in patients ages 10 to 40 years old.

■ Other Imaging Findings

- The classic location of a branchial cleft cyst is at the anteromedial border of the sternocleidomastoid muscle (SCM), lateral to the carotid space, and at the posterior margin of the submandibular gland.

- Branchial cleft cysts typically displace the SCM posteriorly or posterolaterally. The vessels of the carotid space are medially or posteromedially displaced and the submandibular gland is anteriorly displaced.
- A thickened wall may indicate infection.
- Depending on mucoid content of the cyst, it may have internal echogenicity and may have increased T1 signal.

✓ Pearls and ✗ Pitfalls

- ✓ A curved rim of tissue may be seen pointing medially between the internal and external carotid arteries. This is referred to as the "beak sign" or "notch sign" and is considered pathognomonic of a second branchial cleft cyst (type III), although a schwannoma can have this finding as well.
- ✓ Branchial cleft fistulae and sinuses can also occur. There may be an obvious opening in the neck between the hyoid bone and suprasternal notch.
- ✗ Although the angle of the mandible is the most frequent location, branchial cleft cysts can occur anywhere along a line from the oropharyngeal tonsillar fossa to the supraclavicular region.

Case 11

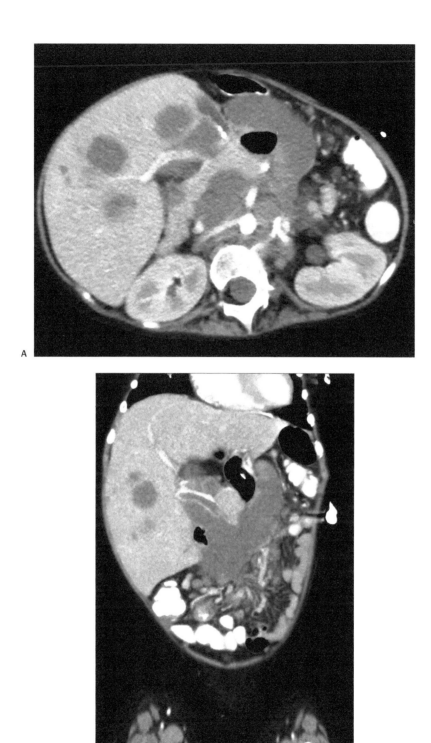

■ Clinical Presentation

A 6-year-old girl with a history of heterotaxy and cardiac transplant presents with abdominal pain and mass.

■ Imaging Findings

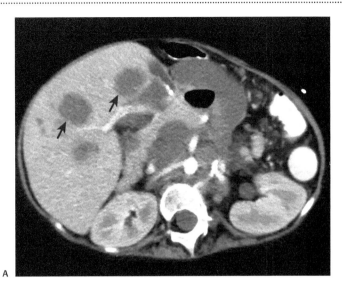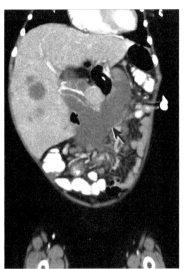

(A) Axial postcontrast CT image demonstrates multiple low-density nodules in the liver (*arrows*), porta hepatis, and around the aortic axis. **(B)** Coronal postcontrast CT image demonstrates the liver and porta hepatis low-density lesions, as well as an elongated mass anterior to the vascular axis (*arrow*).

■ Differential Diagnosis

- ***Posttransplant lymphoproliferative disorder:***
  Given the history of heart transplant and associated immunosuppression, the findings here are most suspicious for posttransplant lymphoproliferative disorder; reducing immunosuppression often brings about remission.
- *Lymphoma:* Lymphoma is part of a spectrum of lymphoproliferative diseases that includes posttransplant lymphoproliferative disorder, and the two can be very difficult to distinguish; patients after heart transplant have a relatively high incidence.
- *Granulomatous disease:* Infectious diseases such as cat-scratch disease and mononucleosis (which, like posttransplant lymphoproliferative disorder, is linked to Epstein–Barr virus) can be associated with prominent and confluent lymphadenopathy.

■ Essential Facts

- Patients present with lymphadenopathy and associated mass effect.
- Enlarged nodes can be found anywhere in the body but most often in the abdomen.
- More common in children than in adults.

■ Other Imaging Findings

- Bowel wall thickening that can precipitate intussusception.
- May see diffuse involvement and enlargement of the spleen.
- Positron emission tomography (PET) and PET/CT can be useful for determining extent of disease and response to therapy.

✓ Pearls and ✗ Pitfalls

✓ Posttransplant lymphoproliferative disease is the presumptive diagnosis in a posttransplant patient on immunosuppression who develops prominent adenopathy and/or mass.

✗ Risk of posttransplant lymphoproliferative disorder is highest in children who are Epstein-Barr negative at time of transplant and become infected thereafter.

Case 12

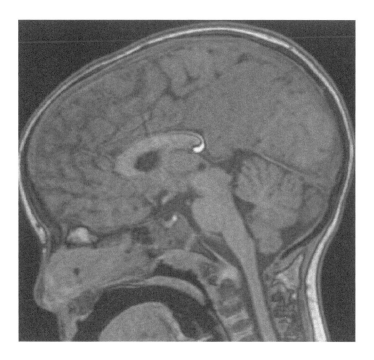

■ Clinical Presentation

A 3-year-old boy with seizures.

■ Imaging Findings

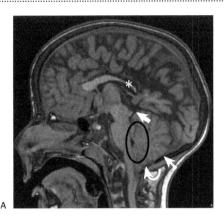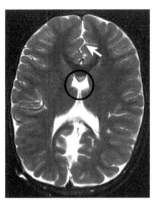

(A) Sagittal T1 noncontrast MR image. The posterior fossa is small (*thin arrow*) and the cerebellum is herniated through the foramen magnum (*curved arrow*). The fourth ventricle is small and there is aqueductal stenosis (*circle*). There is tectal beaking (*thick arrow*). Hypoplasia/agenesis of the posterior body of the corpus callosum (*asterisk*) is seen. **(B)** Axial T2 fat-saturated noncontrast MR image. There is interdigitation of the falx (*arrow*) and the septum pellucidum is not identified (*circle*).

■ Differential Diagnosis

- **Chiari II malformation:** The constellation of findings as well as the history of myelomeningocele make this the most likely diagnosis.
- *Chiari I malformation:* In this malformation, the cerebellar tonsils are displaced > 5 mm caudally through the foramen magnum; however, there usually are no other cerebral abnormalities and it is not associated with myelomeningocele, although it is associated with syringomyelia.
- *Chiari III malformation:* Features of Chiari II overlap with Chiari III; however, in Chiari III, the posterior fossa contents herniate into an occipital or high cervical cephalocele.

■ Essential Facts

- Chiari II malformation is characterized by a myelomeningocele and a small posterior fossa with the medulla and fourth ventricle being inferiorly displaced and the cerebellum herniating through the foramen magnum.
- Hydrocephalus often requires shunting.
- Also called Arnold–Chiari malformation.

■ Other Imaging Findings

- Supratentorially: Enlarged massa intermedia, colpocephaly, hydrocephalus.
- Infratentorially: Petrous bone scalloping, low torcula, cervicomedullary kinking.
- Spinal dysraphism such as meningocele, myelomeningocele, tethered cord, filum lipoma.
- Lacunar skull (Lückenschädel skull): Round or ovoid pits on the inner surface of the skull that are separated by ridges of bone.

✓ Pearls and ✗ Pitfalls

- ✓ Lemon sign. On prenatal ultrasound image, there is indentation of the frontal bone that makes the skull appear to be lemon shaped.
- ✓ Banana sign. On axial images through the posterior fossa on prenatal ultrasound, the cerebellum is wrapped around the brainstem, and the cerebellum looks like a banana.
- ✗ Lacunar skull (Lückenschädel skull) finding disappears after 6 months of age.
- ✗ Lemon skull sign is most frequently seen in fetuses < 24 weeks' gestational age and may not be present in older fetuses. It is not exclusive to Chiari II and can be seen in fetuses with encephaloceles and other conditions.

Case 14

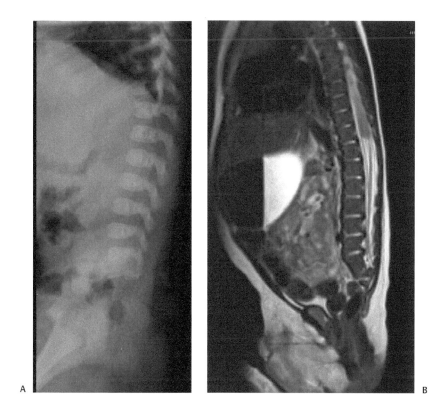

A

B

▦ Clinical Presentation

A newborn with a large sacral dimple.

■ Imaging Findings

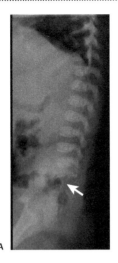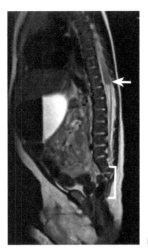

A   B

(A) Lateral X-ray of the lumbar spine. The sacrum and coccyx are not identified (*arrow*). (B) Sagittal T2-weighted MR image of the spine. The conus medullaris (*arrow*) is blunted and located at the T11–T12 level. There is absence of the sacrum and coccyx (*bracket*).

■ Differential Diagnosis

- **Caudal regression syndrome (CRS):** Sacral agenesis with a truncated, blunt spinal cord with a high termination is consistent with CRS.
- *Currarino triad:* There is a sacrococcygeal defect; however, there is no anorectal malformation or presacral mass as would be needed to complete the Currarino triad.
- *Sirenomelia:* Although this patient has sacrococcygeal agenesis, she does not have the other findings of lower limb fusion, anorectal atresia, and genitourinary abnormalities. Furthermore, this is a fatal congenital defect and survival at birth is rare.

■ Essential Facts

- CRS is a congenital abnormality in which a portion of the lumbosacral spine and spinal cord fails to develop. Abnormalities range from partial agenesis of the coccyx to agenesis of the lumbar spine or sacrum.
- CRS is associated with other congenital anomalies, especially of the gastrointestinal and genitourinary systems.

■ Other Imaging Findings

- The most characteristic feature of the spinal cord is the wedge-shaped spinal cord terminus—the dorsal aspect extends more caudally than the ventral portion.
- The spinal cord ends more superiorly than is expected.
- Skeletal findings: Dysraphic/dysplastic vertebral defects, hip dislocation/dysplasia, clubfoot, narrow pelvis.
- Genitourinary findings: Renal dysplasia/agenesis, hydronephrosis, renal ectopia.
- Gastrointestinal findings: Imperforate anus or anorectal atresia, esophageal or duodenal atresia.

✓ Pearls and ✗ Pitfalls

- ✓ May be associated with VACTERL (vertebral defects, anal atresia, cardiac defects, tracheoesophageal fistula, renal anomalies, and limb abnormalities) syndrome.
- ✗ The spinal cord may be tethered despite the location of the conus.

Case 15

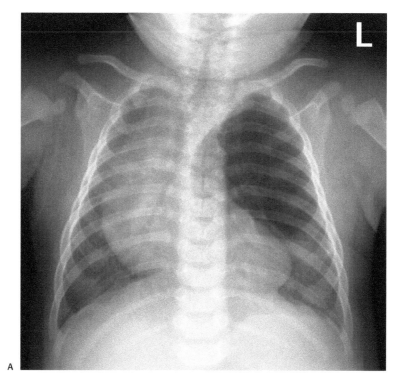

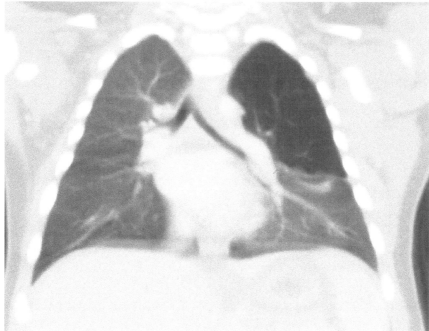

■ Clinical Presentation

A 4-month-old with respiratory distress.

■ Imaging Findings

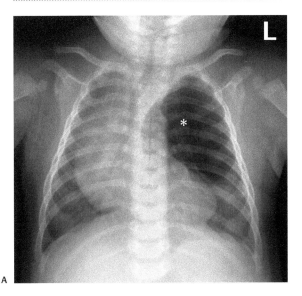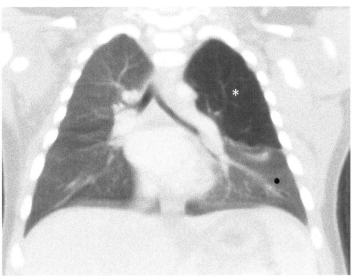

(A) Anteroposterior X-ray of the chest. Hyperexpansion of the left upper lobe (*asterisk*) is seen with displacement of the mediastinum to the right. **(B)** Coronal CT image of the chest. The left upper lobe (*asterisk*) is hyperinflated with vascular attenuation. The lower lobe (*dot*) is mildly compressed.

■ Differential Diagnosis

- **Congenital lobar overinflation:** Hyperinflation of the left upper lobe is typical of congenital lobar emphysema.
- *Congenital bronchial atresia:* Although hyperinflation and vascular attenuation is seen, there is no tubular soft tissue structure consistent with a mucocele.
- *Congenital pulmonary airway malformation (CPAM):* These are multicystic air-filled lesions. These can be large lesions leading to mass effect and mediastinal shift; however, the cysts should displace the vascularity, whereas this lesion has vascularity running through it.

■ Essential Facts

- Congenital lobar overinflation is also called *congenital lobar emphysema.*
- Patients are typically newborns with respiratory distress; however, it can present as late as 6 months of age.
- May be associated with cardiovascular anomalies in up to 15% of cases.

■ Other Imaging Findings

- At birth, the affected lobe can be opaque and homogeneous due to retained fetal fluid. Alternatively, distended lymphatic channels resorbing the fetal fluid may appear as a diffuse reticular pattern.
- May appear as a unilateral hyperlucent hemithorax.
- Decubitus films may be helpful to demonstrate air trapping.
- The ipsilateral hemidiaphragm may be depressed, there may be rib space widening, and the affected lobe may herniate across the mediastinum.
- On fetal ultrasound image, these may appear as a homogeneously hyperechoic mass.

✓ Pearls and ✗ Pitfalls

- ✓ Most commonly affected lobes are left upper, right middle, and then right upper.
- ✓ 5% of the time, more than one lobe is involved.
- ✗ The underlying cause can be an intrinsic cartilaginous abnormality; however, extrinsic compression of an airway, such as by a large pulmonary artery or bronchogenic cyst, can also be the culprit.

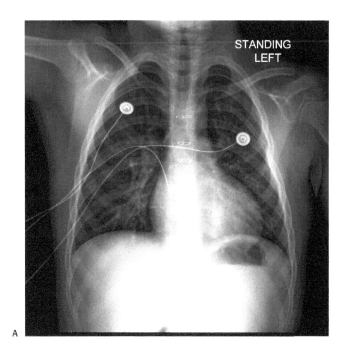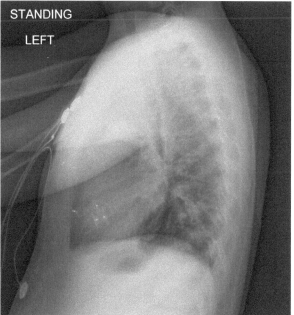

Case 16

■ Clinical Presentation

An 8-year-old boy with a history of ventricular septal defect.

■ Imaging Findings

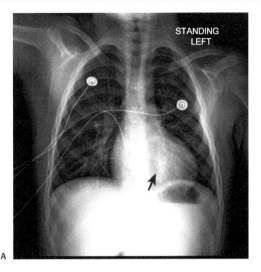 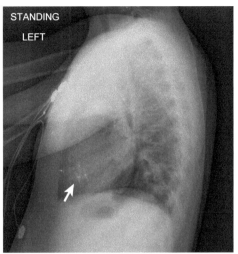

(A) Frontal chest radiograph demonstrates sternotomy wires and two meshlike closure devices superimposed over the expected location of the interventricular septum (*arrow*). **(B)** Lateral chest radiograph better demonstrates the dumbbell shape of the closure devices, which again are superimposed over the interventricular septum (*arrow*).

■ Differential Diagnosis

- ***Ventricular septal defect (VSD) closure device:*** The appearance and location of the object are typical for a VSD closure device.
- *Artifact:* A radiopaque object outside the patient could be mistaken for a closure device, although in this case, the object is superimposed over the heart on two orthogonal views, proving that it is in the heart.
- *Atrial septal defect (ASD) closure device:* An ASD closure device would be located more superiorly and posteriorly than the device in this case.

■ Essential Facts

- Closure devices are available for treatment of VSDs, ASDs, and patent ductus arteriosus.
- Such closure devices are placed using a percutaneous transcatheter technique.
- They are positioned during fluoroscopic and echocardiographic observation.

- They can be repositioned and even removed during the procedure.
- Rates of successful closure with such devices are very high.

■ Other Imaging Findings

- Complications include infection, perforation, malposition, and thrombus formation.

✓ Pearls and ✗ Pitfalls

- ✓ MRI can be safely performed in patients with these devices.
- ✗ Should not be placed in patients with a recent history of sepsis.

Case 17

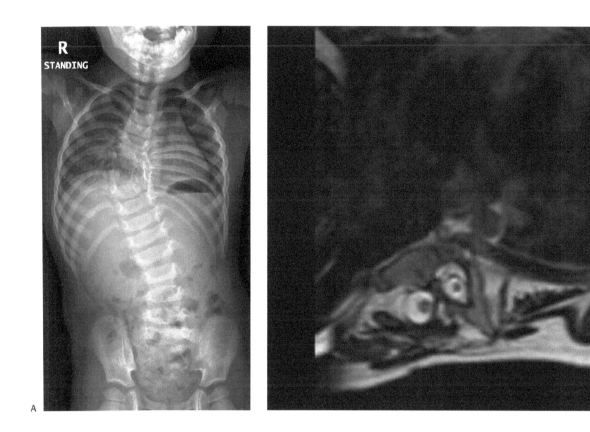

B

■ Clinical Presentation

A 3-year-old girl with scoliosis.

■ Imaging Findings

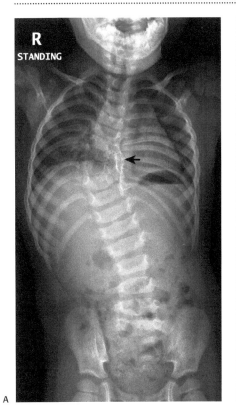
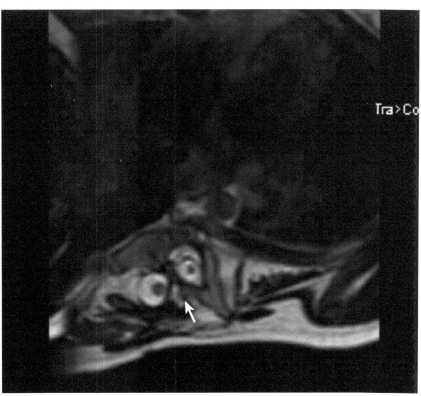

(A) Anteroposterior scoliosis view of the spine. There are segmentation anomalies of the sixth through the ninth vertebral bodies including fusion of the left pedicles (*arrow*) at these levels. There is a C-shaped dextroscoliosis centered at T8. (B) Axial T2-weighted MR image of the midthoracic spine. There is a bony spur (*arrow*) extending through the spinal canal dividing the spinal cord into two separate hemicords, each contained in their own dural sac.

■ Differential Diagnosis

- **Diastematomyelia type 1:** A bony or cartilaginous spur separating two hemicords within their own dural sacs is consistent with type 1 diastematomyelia.
- *Diastematomyelia type 2:* In this condition, there are two hemicords; however, they are within a single dural sac and there is no bony septum. Occasionally, there is a fibrous septum.
- *Diplomyelia:* This refers to a complete duplication of the spinal cord, whereas diastematomyelia refers to a single cord that has been split. Some sources group both together and refer to it as a split cord malformation.

■ Essential Facts

- Type 1 is the classic diastematomyelia that presents with scoliosis and tethered cord syndrome.
- Type 2 is the milder form that may be less symptomatic or even asymptomatic.
- At birth, patients may not have symptoms but later can develop bowel/bladder dysfunction, motor/sensory difficulties, and progressive pain.

■ Other Imaging Findings

- In most cases, the hemicords reunite caudal to the cleft. Occasionally, they do not and there will be two separate conus medullaris.
- Plain radiographs may show widening of the spinal canal, vertebral anomalies, scoliosis, and perhaps a midline bony ridge.
- Axial ultrasound images typically demonstrate both hemicords in cross section, each with a central canal and nerve roots.
- Ultrasound may demonstrate associated malformations such as syringomyelia or thickened filum terminalis.

✓ Pearls and ✕ Pitfalls

- ✓ A hairy tuft on the patient's back can sometimes be seen on physical exam.
- ✓ Prenatal ultrasound image may show the abnormality.
- ✓ Diastematomyelia is rare in the cervical cord.
- ✕ If there is an osseous septum separating the hemicords, the shadow from the bone usually makes ultrasound examination of the spinal cord nearly impossible at that level.

Case 18

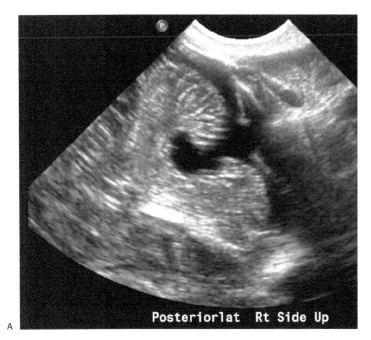

Posteriorlat   Rt Side Up

A

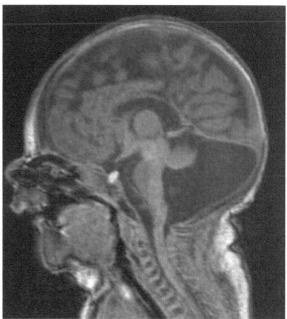

B

■ Clinical Presentation

A newborn with macrocephaly.

■ Imaging Findings

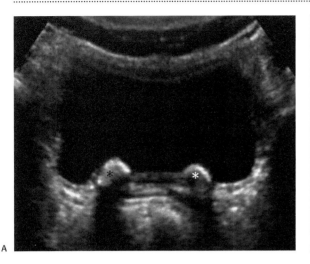
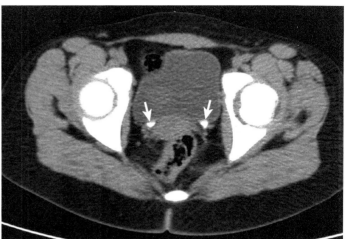

(A) Transverse ultrasound image of the bladder. There are round, shadowing, echogenic masses (*asterisks*) along the posterior bladder wall at the ureterovesical junctions (UVJs). **(B)** Axial noncontrast CT image of the pelvis. There are round, high-density masses (*arrows*) at the UVJs.

■ Differential Diagnosis

- ***Deflux injections:*** Round, hyperechoic, shadowing masses on ultrasound image at the bilateral ureterovesical junctions (UVJs) that correspond with calcified masses on CT image are consistent with Deflux (Oceana Therapeutics, Edison, NJ) injections for the treatment of vesicoureteral reflux (VUR).
- *Stones lodged at the ureterovesical junctions:* Although it would be unusual for a patient to have bilateral stones at the UVJ, it could happen. With stones this large, there would be hydroureteronephrosis and a history of pain. For ultrasound, the patient could be placed in the decubitus position to see whether the stones layer in the dependent portion of the bladder in order to exclude stones that have already passed.
- *Bladder rhabdomyosarcoma:* This usually appears as a heterogeneous mass with both solid and cystic components. Patients usually present with hematuria and/or dysuria.

■ Essential Facts

- Deflux, a dextranomer–hyaluronic acid copolymer made by Oceana Therapeutics, is used as a bulking agent at the VUJ for the endoscopic treatment of VUR.
- Approximately 1.0 to 1.5 mL of Deflux is injected per ureter.
- Polytef (Teflon, DuPont, Wilmington, DE) and silicone are no longer used because of the propensity to migrate to distant organs and to form granulomas.
- Cure rates of endoscopic treatment for VUR have significantly improved, rivaling those of open ureteral reimplantation.

■ Other Imaging Findings

- Deflux has a radiographic appearance consistent with soft tissue, so initially it is not seen on plain films. It may, however, calcify several years after injection and appear on plain films.
- Deflux injections may appear as calcified or noncalcified on CT.
- On MRI, Deflux injections are bright on T2 imaging and are not seen on T1-weighted imaging. They do not enhance with gadolinium.

✓ Pearls and ✗ Pitfalls

✓ The patient's history can help to distinguish calcified Deflux injections from stones. The side of the injection and flank pain, the presence of hydronephrosis and hematuria, and the exact location of calcification in relation to the ureterovesical junction can be distinguishing factors.

✗ Deflux injections may change in size over time and may become less visible on imaging.

Case 20

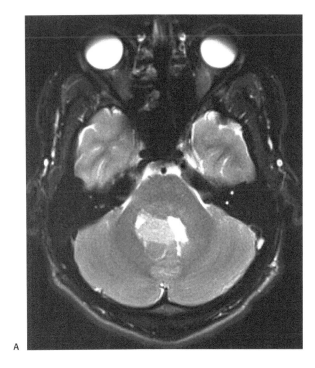

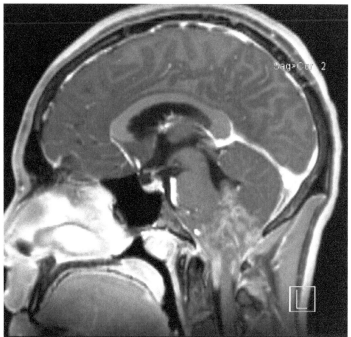

A

B

▦ Clinical Presentation

A 16-year-old boy with intermittent headaches.

■ Imaging Findings

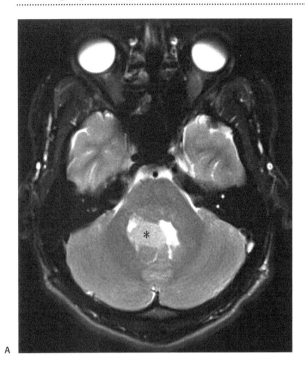
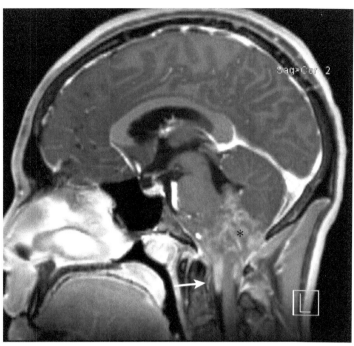

(A) Axial T2 fat-saturated image of the brain. There is a soft tissue mass (*asterisk*) originating from the right side of the fourth ventricle. **(B)** Sagittal T1 postcontrast. There is a heterogeneously enhancing mass (*asterisk*) that extends inferiorly through the foramen magnum and into the cervical spinal canal (*arrow*).

■ Differential Diagnosis

- **Ependymoma:** This is a soft or "plastic" tumor that arises in the fourth ventricle and extends through the foramina into the cisterns.
- *Medulloblastoma:* This also arises in the fourth ventricle; however, it expands the ventricle rather than escaping through the foramina.
- *Brainstem glioma:* This is also a common pediatric infratentorial neoplasm; however, this is an infiltrating tumor that expands the brainstem.

■ Essential Facts

- Although the most common location is within the fourth ventricle, ependymomas can also arise supratentorially and in the spine, although both of those locations are more frequent in adults.
- Ependymomas are much less common than medulloblastoma or pilocytic astrocytoma.

■ Other Imaging Findings

- Calcification is common.
- Hydrocephalus is almost always present when it occurs in the fourth ventricle.

✓ Pearls and ✗ Pitfalls

✓ Ependymomas have an indistinct interface with the floor of the fourth ventricle. Medulloblastoma is associated with the roof of the fourth ventricle.

✗ Choroid plexus papillomas can also occur as a lobular mass in the fourth ventricle; however, they are densely enhancing.

Case 21

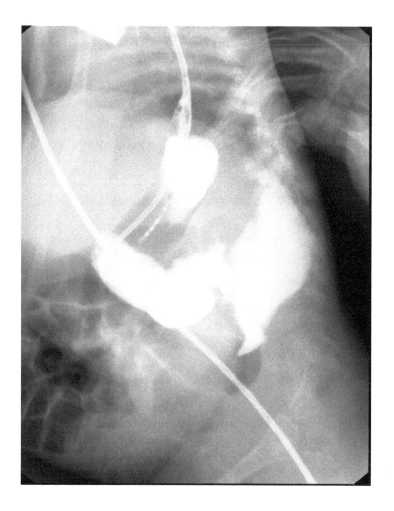

■ Clinical Presentation

A 5-year-old presents with severe abdominal pain.

■ Imaging Findings

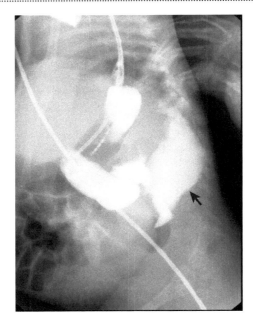

(A) A right-side-down lateral radiograph from an upper gastrointestinal examination with water-soluble contrast demonstrates a large pool of contrast connected to the posterior wall of the second portion of the duodenum (*arrow*).

■ Differential Diagnosis

- **Duodenal perforation:** Leakage of contrast into the peritoneal cavity, or as in this case, the retroperitoneal space behind the descending duodenum, is essentially diagnostic of duodenal perforation.
- *Duodenal diverticulum:* Duodenal diverticula are associated with extension of contrast beyond the expected margins of the duodenal lumen, but diverticula generally have an ovoid shape and smooth, regular walls.
- *Superimposition of other contrast-opacified bowel:* In some cases, the presence of other contrast-pacified segments of bowel can mimic a perforation.

■ Essential Facts

- Perforated peptic ulcers are not common in children.
- Perforation is usually an indication for urgent surgery.
- Complications include peritonitis, sepsis, and death.

■ Other Imaging Findings

- Bowel perforation can be associated with small quantities of extraluminal gas or frank pneumoperitoneum.
- The presence of contrast material in the gut lumen is helpful in such cases, because it renders the location and size of the perforation easy to visualize.
- In cases of nontraumatic perforation, lesions associated with the perforation, such as ulcerations, may be visualized.

✓ Pearls and ✗ Pitfalls

✓ In general, CT is the best examination for evaluating suspected duodenal injury.
✗ Barium contrast should be avoided—it may interfere with subsequent imaging, and spillage can cause peritonitis.
✗ To ensure that other segments of contrast-opacified bowel are not mistaken for perforation, it is important to obtain precontrast images to rule out the presence of retained contrast and also to obtain images in various projections, which should make it possible to distinguish perforation from contrast in other parts of the gastrointestinal tract.

Case 22

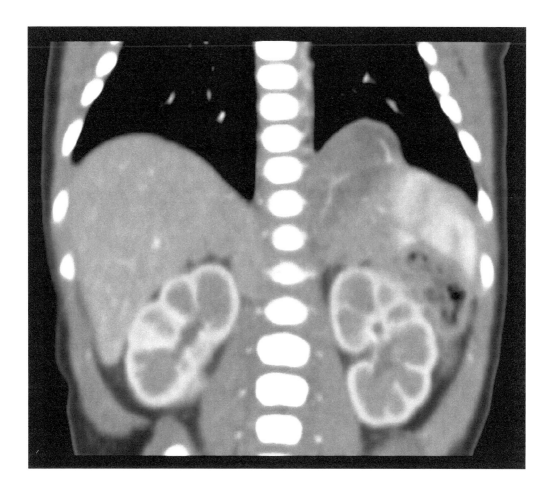

■ Clinical Presentation

A 2-day-old girl with a mass superior to the left kidney seen on prenatal ultrasound image.

■ Imaging Findings

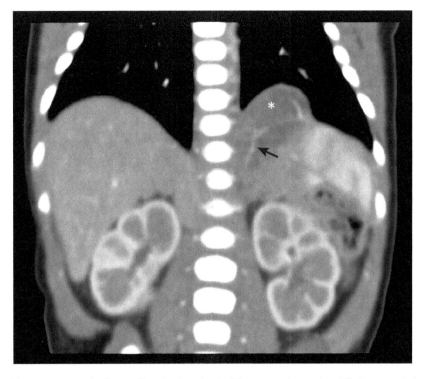

(A) CT image of the chest with contrast, coronal reformat. There is a low-density left suprarenal mass (*asterisk*). It appears to be covered by the left hemidiaphragm and has a large central vessel directed toward the aorta (*arrow*).

■ Differential Diagnosis

- ***Extralobar sequestration:*** An infradiaphragmatic mass with a feeding vessel directed toward the aorta is suspicious for an extralobar sequestration. If the vessel had been shown to originate from the aorta, the diagnosis would have been confirmed.
- *Neuroblastoma:* The location of this lesion would be typical; however, neuroblastoma is more heterogeneous and infiltrative.
- *Lipoid pneumonia:* Although lipoid pneumonia is low density, it would not be found below the hemidiaphragm and would not contain a feeding vessel.

■ Essential Facts

- Sequestration is an area of abnormal lung that does not communicate with the bronchial tree or pulmonary arteries. Sequestrations are nonfunctioning and prone to infection.
- Extralobar sequestration has its own pleural covering and its venous drainage is usually via the systemic veins.

■ Other Imaging Findings

- Does not contain air unless infected.
- On X-ray, it appears as a basilar opacity that is stable over multiple radiographs.
- On contrast-enhanced CT/CT angiography image, a feeding systemic vessel should be identified to confirm the diagnosis.

✓ Pearls and ✗ Pitfalls

- ✓ Systemic vascular supply is typically from the descending aorta; however, it also can arise from the upper abdominal branches of the aorta.
- ✗ It can be very difficult to distinguish intralobar sequestration from extralobar sequestration.

Case 23

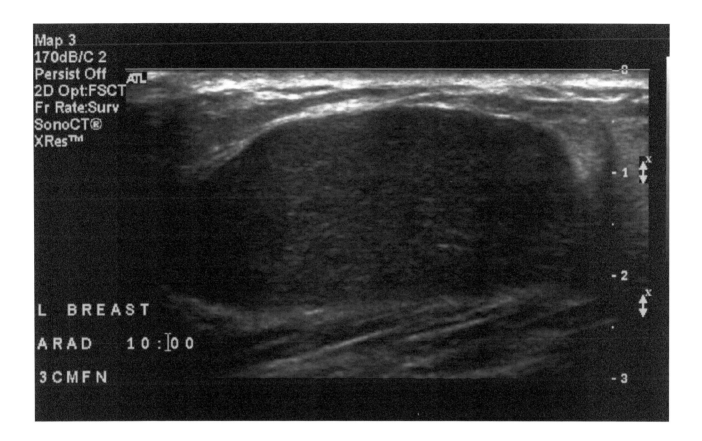

■ Clinical Presentation

A 12-year-old girl with a palpable mass in the upper outer quadrant of the left breast.

■ Imaging Findings

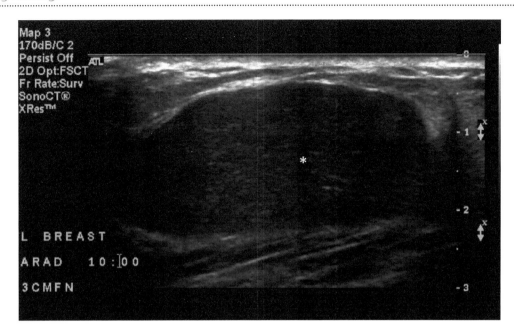

(A) Transverse grayscale ultrasound view of the left breast. In the left breast, there is a well-circumscribed, homogeneous, hypoechoic ovoid mass without through transmission (*asterisk*). The long axis of the mass is parallel to the chest wall.

■ Differential Diagnosis

- **Fibroadenoma:** The characteristics of this mass in a young girl are compatible with fibroadenoma.
- *Phyllodes tumor:* The imaging appearance of phyllodes tumor is similar to fibroadenoma, and a true distinction of the two can only be made by biopsy. The internal architecture of phyllodes tumor is more frequently heterogeneous when compared to fibroadenomas, and phyllodes tumors often contain anechoic cysts or clefts.
- *Complex fibroadenoma:* These contain cysts, sclerosing adenosis, epithelial calcifications, or areas of papillary apocrine metaplasia. Typically seen in older patients.

■ Essential Facts

- Fibroadenomas are benign masses caused by overgrowth of the connective tissue stroma of the breast lobule.
- Painless, mobile, "rubbery" masses.
- Most often located in the upper outer quadrant.

■ Other Imaging Findings

- Can range in size from microscopic to large and can be single or multiple.
- On ultrasound, they are round, oval, or macrolobulated, well-circumscribed, and uniformly hypoechoic masses, although they may appear anechoic with low-level internal echoes.

- There is an abrupt interface between the lesion and normal breast tissue with variable posterior acoustic transmission.
- Avascular or mildly increased blood flow.
- Long axis is parallel to the chest wall.
- Mammography is not typically used in children, but fibroadenomas appear as well-defined, round, oval, or macrolobulated masses with popcornlike calcifications.
- Fibroadenomas can be incidentally seen on CT. They appear as well-demarcated, ovoid, round, or smoothly lobulated noncalcified masses.

✓ Pearls and ✗ Pitfalls

✓ Most common breast mass in girls younger than 19 years of age.
✓ Generally not seen before puberty.
✓ 10% regress spontaneously.
✓ A subtype of fibroadenoma called a juvenile or cellular fibroadenoma frequently undergoes rapid growth and occurs most often in African American girls.
✗ Management is controversial. Some recommend short-term follow-up; others recommend biopsy.
✗ Adolescents with complex fibroadenomas are at a slightly higher risk of developing breast cancer.
✗ Fibroadenomas have a variable appearance on MR image, and MRI cannot differentiate them from phyllodes tumors.

Case 24

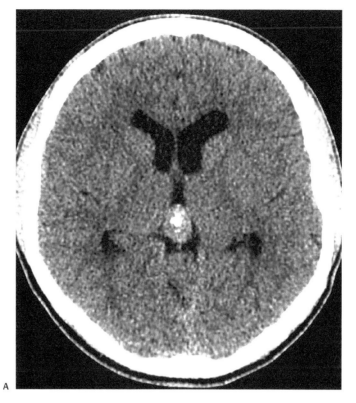

A

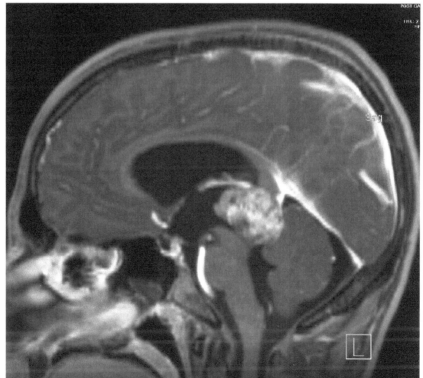

B

A 17-year-old boy with diabetes insipidus.

■ Imaging Findings

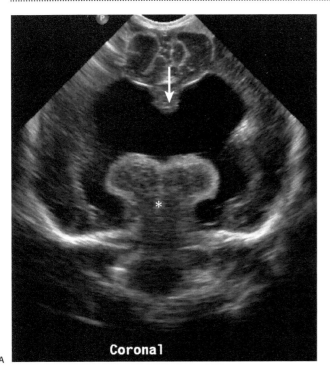

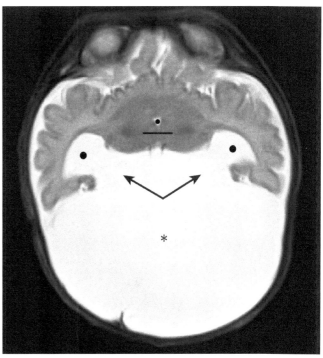

(A) Coronal grayscale ultrasound image of the head. There is absence of the septum pellucidum with fusion of the lateral ventricles (*arrow*). The thalami are fused (*asterisk*). (B) Axial T2-weighted image of the brain. There is a large cerebrospinal fluid–filled dorsal cyst (*asterisk*) communicating with a large monoventricle (*arrows*). The temporal horns are partially formed (*dots*). The dorsal cyst severely anteriorly displaces and compresses the cerebral parenchyma. The basal ganglia are partially fused anteriorly (*line*). There is a small third ventricle (*small dot*). Again noted is absence of the septum pellucidum.

■ Differential Diagnosis

- **Holoprosencephaly (severe semilobar):** A large monoventricle communicating with a dorsal cyst with partially fused basal ganglia and a small third ventricle is consistent with this diagnosis.
- *Severe hydrocephalus:* In severe hydrocephalus, there should be a thin rim of cortex surrounding the massively dilated ventricles. In addition, the midline structures including the septum pellucidum should be present and there should not be fusion of the basal ganglia.
- *Hydranencephaly:* In hydranencephaly, the remaining cerebral cortex should be along the tentorium and the parenchyma in the carotid distribution should be obliterated.

■ Essential Facts

- Holoprosencephaly is a spectrum with congenital forebrain abnormality characterized by the lack of development of the midline structures.

■ Other Imaging Findings

- Alobar holoprosencephaly: Most severe. Single, midline monoventricle with pancake-shaped anterior cerebral tissue and fusion of the thalami. The corpus callosum, interhemispheric fissure, cavum septum pellucidum, and third ventricle are absent.
- Semilobar holoprosencephaly: The septum pellucidum is absent. There is a monoventricle with partially developed temporal and occipital horns and an incompletely formed interhemispheric fissure. There is partial or complete fusion of the thalami with agenesis or partial agenesis of the corpus callosum.
- Lobar holoprosencephaly: Least severe. There is fusion of the frontal horns of the lateral ventricles, which widely communicate with the third ventricle. There is absence of the septum pellucidum, but the corpus callosum can be normal or hypoplastic.

✓ Pearls and ✗ Pitfalls

✓ Midline facial anomalies associated with holoprosencephaly are also a spectrum, with the most severe associated with alobar holoprosencephaly. Patients with the lobar type may have no facial anomaly.

✗ Because holoprosencephaly is a spectrum, some patients may have findings on the border between types.

Case 26

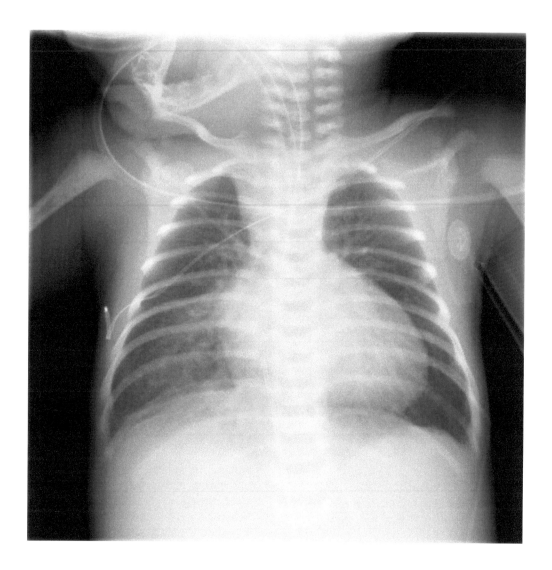

■ Clinical Presentation

A 2-day-old boy with cyanosis and respiratory distress.

■ Imaging Findings

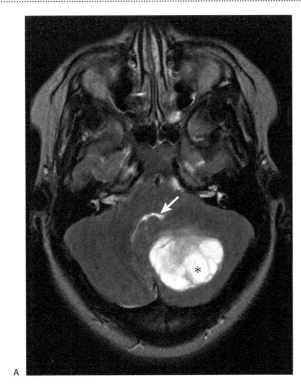 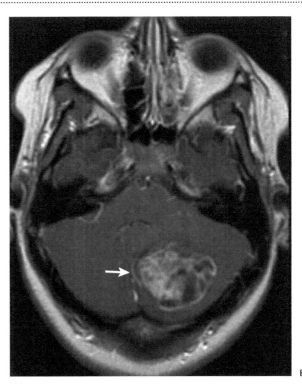

(A) Axial T2 MR image with fat saturation. There is a complex cystic mass in the left cerebellar hemisphere (*asterisk*) that causes effacement of the fourth ventricle (*arrow*). **(B)** Axial T1 MR image postcontrast. The solid components of the mass enhance (*arrow*).

■ Differential Diagnosis

- ***Juvenile pilocytic astrocytoma (JPA):*** The cystic and solid appearance, location, and enhancement pattern are typical of an astrocytoma.
- *Medulloblastoma*: These dense tumors arise from the roof of the fourth ventricle.
- *Ependymoma:* These usually fill the fourth ventricle and can extend into the cerebellopontine angle.

■ Essential Facts

- Pilocytic astrocytoma is the most common pediatric cerebellar neoplasm.
- The overall prognosis of patients with pilocytic astrocytoma is excellent, especially if there is complete resection. Pilocytic astrocytomas in the optic chiasm/ hypothalamic region have the least favorable prognosis of all locations.

■ Other Imaging Findings

- Most of these tumors are round or oval and have well-circumscribed, smooth margins. They are often mixed cystic and solid and have occasional calcifications.
- Most have intense contrast enhancement.
- Distant dissemination is rare.

✓ Pearls and ✗ Pitfalls

✓ Two thirds of JPAs have the classic imaging presentation of a cystlike mass with an enhancing mural nodule.
✗ In children, the most common location for pilocytic astrocytoma is in the cerebellum; however, in adults, it is the cerebral hemispheres.

Case 34

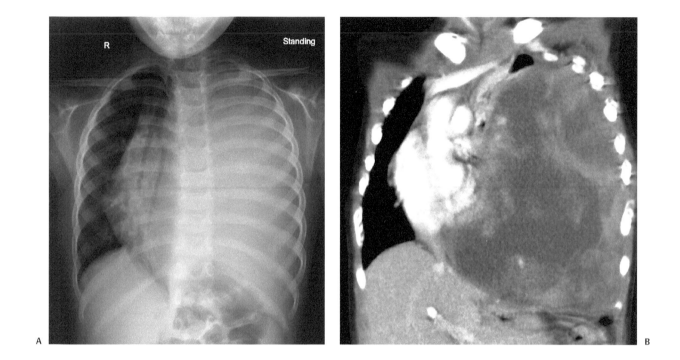

■ Clinical Presentation

....

A 4-year-old girl with fever and cough.

▣ Imaging Findings

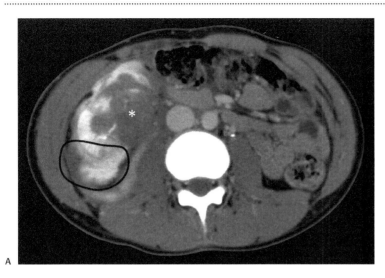 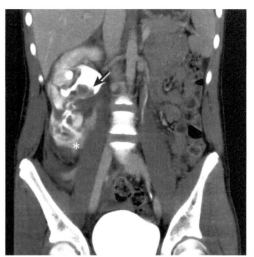

(A) Axial postcontrast CT image of the abdomen. In the lower pole of the right kidney, there is low density extending through the anterior renal cortex (*asterisk*). In addition, there is extravasated contrast and fluid surrounding the kidney (*circle*). **(B)** Coronal postcontrast CT image of the abdomen. Again, low density is seen extending through the renal cortex into the collecting system with extravasation of contrast (*asterisk*). Within the renal collecting system, there is round, masslike low density displacing the excreted contrast in the collecting system (*arrow*).

▣ Differential Diagnosis

- ***Grade IV renal laceration:*** When a renal laceration extends to the renal pelvis and there is urinary and contrast extravasation, this is consistent with a grade IV laceration. There is a thrombus in the collecting system.
- *Grade III renal laceration:* Grade III renal lacerations do not extend to the renal pelvis or collecting system and extravasation of urine or contrast should not be identified.
- *Grade V renal laceration*: Grade V renal laceration consists of a completely shattered kidney with devascularization of the kidney due to avulsion of the renal hilum.

▣ Essential Facts

- The American Association for the Surgery of Trauma (AAST) renal injury scale predicts the need for kidney repair, removal, morbidity, and mortality after renal injuries.
- Grade I renal injury consists of a subcapsular, nonexpanding hematoma without a parenchymal laceration.
- Grade II renal injury consists of a nonexpanding perirenal hematoma confined to the retroperitoneum and/or a parenchymal laceration of < 1 cm depth without urinary extravasation.
- When assigning an AAST grade, advance one grade for bilateral injuries up to grade III.
- Renal CT is indicated in trauma patients with gross hematuria, contusion or hematoma of the soft tissues of the flank, hypotension, lumbar spinal injury, and fractures of the lower ribs or a transverse process.

▣ Other Imaging Findings

- Contrast-enhanced multidetector CT is the modality of choice for imaging renal trauma because it assesses the renal parenchyma, collecting system, and vascularity.
- Ultrasound may be helpful in diagnosing hemoperitoneum, but it is not as sensitive as CT for diagnosing parenchymal injuries.
- If renal injury is detected on a trauma portal venous phase CT image without evidence of extravasation, then a 5- to 15-minute delayed phase series should be considered to assess for urine extravasation, especially if there are clinical signs of collecting system injury.
- The most common complication is urinoma. Delayed bleeding can occur 1 to 2 weeks after the trauma.

✓ Pearls and ✗ Pitfalls

- ✓ Children with blunt trauma should undergo renal imaging regardless of the presence of hypotension or the degree of hematuria.
- ✓ The incidence of renal injures increases in preexisting congenital or acquired renal pathology such as cysts, tumors, chronic hydronephrosis, and congenital anomalies such as a horseshoe kidney, ectopic kidney, congenital ureteropelvic junction obstruction, and polycystic kidneys.
- ✗ Although gross hematuria is the most reliable indicator of serious urologic injury, the degree of hematuria does not correlate with the degree of renal injury.
- ✗ The absence of hematuria does not preclude renal injury.

Case 40

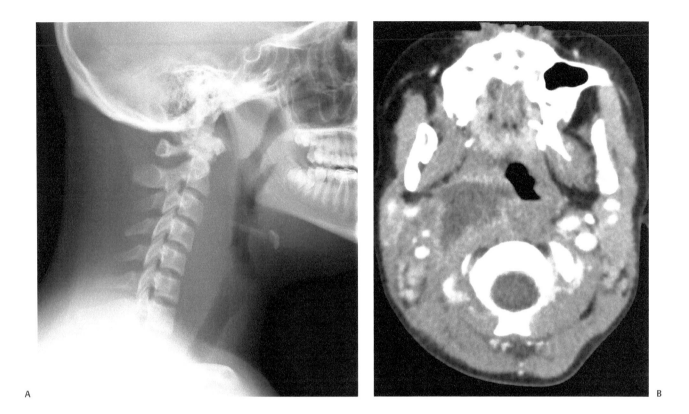

A   B

▦ Clinical Presentation

A 13-year-old boy with sore throat.

■ Imaging Findings

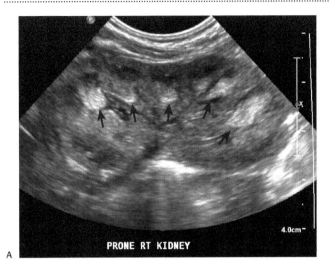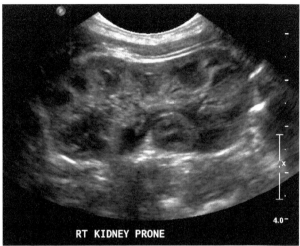

(A) Longitudinal ultrasound image of the right kidney 2 days after birth. The apex of the renal pyramids (papillae) are echogenic (*arrows*). (B) Longitudinal ultrasound image of the right kidney 2 weeks later. The echogenicity at the tips of the renal pyramids has resolved.

■ Differential Diagnosis

- ***Transient hyperechogenicity of the pyramids in neonates and infants (Tamm–Horsfall proteinuria):*** Transient increase in the echogenicity of the renal pyramids in an otherwise healthy newborn that resolves without treatment is consistent with Tamm–Horsfall proteinuria.
- *Candida infection:* This can be difficult to distinguish from Tamm–Horsfall proteinuria because it can cause hyperechogenicity of the papillae, especially in a premature infant, who would be more susceptible to infection. Correlation with blood and urine cultures is helpful. In addition, the natural progression of *Candida* infection would not be to resolve, but the papillae may slough and form fungus balls in the collecting system.
- *Renal vein thrombosis:* Although this can cause abnormal echogenicity of the renal pyramids, the renal pyramids are usually heterogeneous and the overall kidney is usually enlarged. Corticomedullary differentiation may be lost.

■ Essential Facts

- The prevalence of hyperechogenicity at the tips of the renal pyramids varies, but it may be seen in up to 50% of normal neonates.

■ Other Imaging Findings

- The maximal hyperechogenicity is at the apex of the renal pyramids. Echogenicity gradually decreases distal to the papillae up to about halfway up the pyramids.
- The base of the pyramid is normal in echogenicity.
- Usually affects multiple pyramids, but may only affect a few or a single pyramid.
- This is a transient finding and should resolve in several days, but it may take up to 14 days or longer in premature infants.
- Hyperechoic debris may also be noted in the collecting system and bladder.

✓ Pearls and ✗ Pitfalls

- ✓ Double parallel linear echogenicities at the base of the renal pyramids represent the arcuate arteries.
- ✗ The cause of the transient hyperechogenicity of the pyramids remains uncertain and somewhat controversial. It has been debated as to whether it is caused by Tamm–Horsfall proteinuria.

Case 44

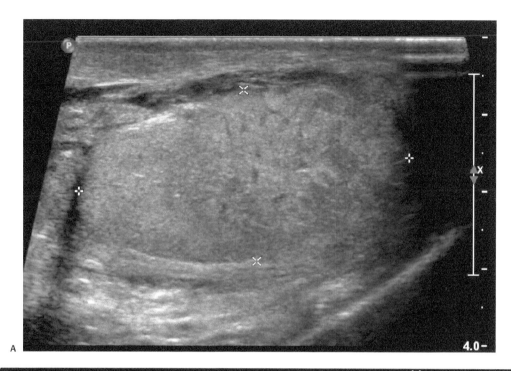

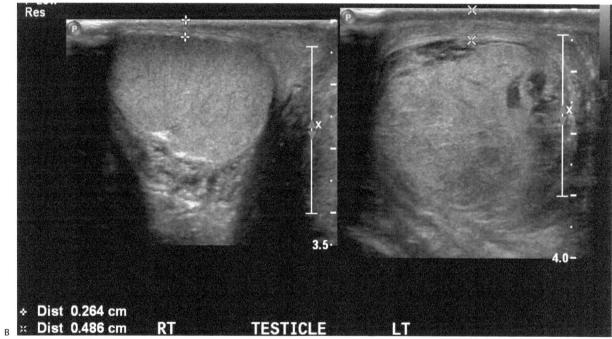

■ Clinical Presentation

A 13-year-old boy with blunt trauma to the scrotum.

■ Imaging Findings

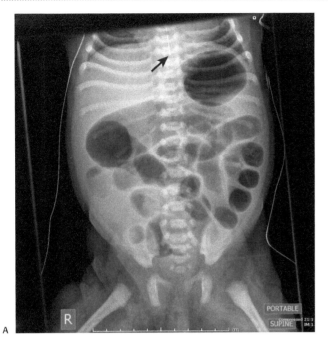 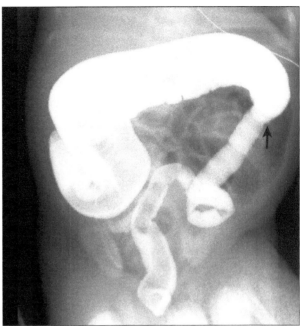

(A) An abdominal radiograph demonstrates many segments of abnormally dilated bowel in a pattern indicating a distal bowel obstruction. An orogastric tube is positioned too high, with its tip in the distal esophagus, where it is unlikely to be effective in decompressing the stomach (*arrow*). **(B)** A radiograph from a contrast enema demonstrates small caliber of the colon extending from the rectum to the splenic flexure, proximal to which the colon becomes markedly dilated (*arrow*).

■ Differential Diagnosis

- **Meconium plug syndrome:** In meconium plug syndrome, the colon distal to the splenic flexure is small in caliber and the colon proximal to the splenic flexure is dilated, a description that perfectly matches this case.
- *Hirschsprung disease:* The findings here are not typical of Hirschsprung disease, where the transition from dilated proximal colon to small-caliber distal colon typically is found in the rectum or sigmoid colon. However, these findings could represent an atypical appearance of Hirschsprung disease.
- *Ileal atresia:* In ileal atresia, the entire colon should be narrow in caliber with no transition to dilated bowel anywhere in the colon.
- *Meconium ileus:* Again, meconium ileus should demonstrate a complete microcolon.

■ Essential Facts

- Often associated with maternal diabetes or the administration of magnesium sulfate as treatment for preeclampsia.
- Usually resolves spontaneously over 1 to 2 days as the colon begins functioning normally; contrast enema may be helpful in stimulating the colon.
- If obstruction persists, biopsy to rule out Hirschsprung disease.

■ Other Imaging Findings

- The rectum is usually larger in caliber than the sigmoid colon, arguing against Hirschsprung disease.
- The point of transition in colon caliber does not need to be exactly at the splenic flexure.

✓ Pearls and ✗ Pitfalls

- ✓ On contrast enema, once the point of transition in colon caliber is identified, there is no need to reflux contrast more proximally.
- ✓ Patience may be required to reflux contrast past meconium plugs in the distal colon.
- ✗ Imaging findings cannot exclude an atypical appearance of Hirschsprung disease, which should be suspected if the patient fails to improve over 1 to 2 days.

Case 47

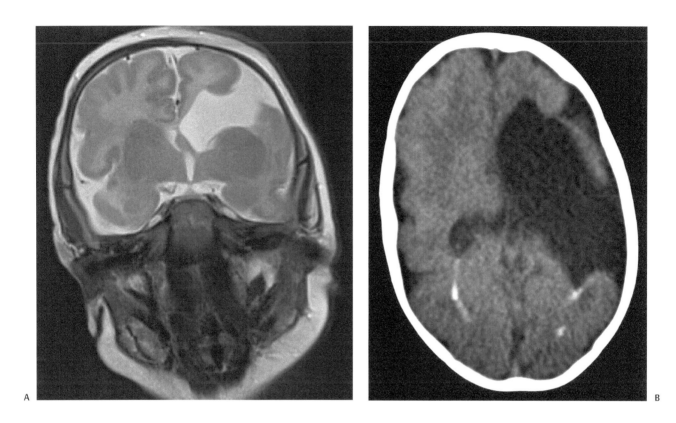

A   B

A 5-month-old with a history of congenital microcephaly.

■ Imaging Findings

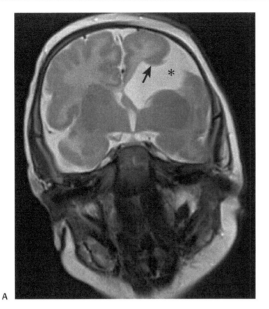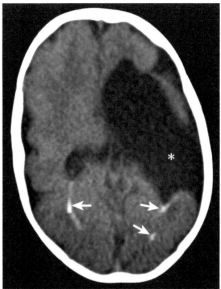

A   B

(A) Coronal noncontrast T2-weighted MR image of the head. There is a gray matter—lined cleft (*arrow*) that extends from the left lateral ventricle to the extra-axial space (*asterisk*). The walls of the clefts do not touch and are separated by cerebrospinal fluid (open-lipped schizencephaly). **(B)** Axial noncontrast CT image of the head. There are dystrophic calcifications (*arrows*) along the posterior aspects of the lateral ventricles. Again seen is the open-lipped schizencephaly (*asterisk*).

■ Differential Diagnosis

- ***Congenital cytomegalovirus (CMV) infection:*** The findings of disordered migration and periventricular calcifications are consistent with congenital CMV infection.
- *Congenital toxoplasmosis infection:* The calcifications in congenital toxoplasmosis are usually scattered throughout the brain parenchyma instead of being periventricular as in CMV. Congenital toxoplasmosis is much less common than CMV in the United States but is more prevalent in France and Belgium.
- *Congenital rubella or syphilis:* These infections rarely cause brain calcifications.

■ Essential Facts

- Congenital CMV infection is the most common intrauterine infection in the United States and is the most common congenital viral infection in the world.
- CMV is most harmful to the fetus when the mother has a primary infection while pregnant, in which congenital CMV occurs in about one third of patients. The rate of transmission from mother to fetus of a recurrent CMV infection is ~1.5%.

■ Other Imaging Findings

- Neurologic findings can include intracranial calcification, ventriculomegaly, intraventricular adhesions, periventricular cysts, white matter disease, neuronal migrational disorders, and cerebellar hypoplasia and microcephaly.
- Hepatomegaly, splenomegaly.
- Fetal intrahepatic calcification and echogenic bowel.

✓ Pearls and ✗ Pitfalls

- ✓ The different types of congenital infections can be remembered with the mnemonic TORCH: toxoplasmosis; other (syphilis); rubella; cytomegalovirus; herpes.
- ✓ The earlier the gestational age at the time of infection, the more severe the fetal findings.
- ✗ Pseudo-TORCH syndrome (Baraitser–Reardon syndrome) has the same imaging findings as a TORCH infection but with negative serologies.

Case 48

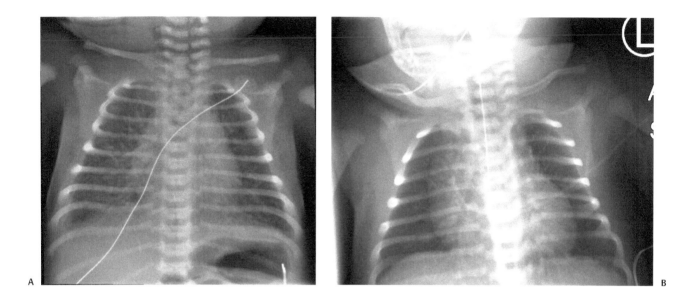

A   B

■ Clinical Presentation

A term newborn with respiratory distress. First image was taken at birth, and the second was taken 36 hours later.

◼ Imaging Findings

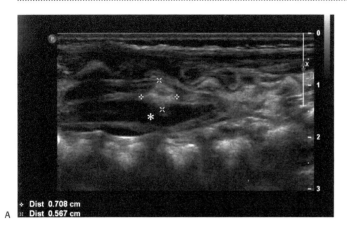
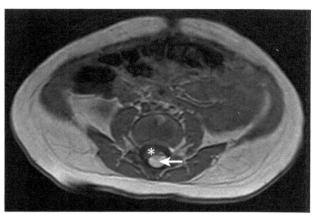

(A) Longitudinal ultrasound view of the lower lumbar spine. There is a subcentimeter echogenic mass (*calipers*) adjacent to the posterior surface of the spinal cord. It displaces the cord (*asterisk*) anteriorly. **(B)** Noncontrast axial T1 volumetric interpolated breath-hold examination MR image of the lumbar spine. There is an ovoid high signal intensity mass (*arrow*) in the left side of the spinal canal that displaces the cord (*asterisk*) to the right. It has the same signal intensity as fat but is not contiguous with the subcutaneous fat.

◼ Differential Diagnosis

- **Intradural lipoma:** The T1 hyperintensity is consistent with fat. The fatty mass does not extend outside of the spinal canal or into the spine itself. No open spinal dysraphism is shown on these images.
- *Lipomyelomeningocele:* In lipomyelomeningocele, the lipoma is adjacent to a cleft in the spinal cord and extends into the central canal of the cord as well as into the spinal canal. The lipoma is continuous with the subcutaneous fat and is covered by intact skin.
- *Fibrolipoma of the filum terminale:* In this situation, the hyperintense T1 signal would be within the filum terminale instead of adjacent to the cord.

◼ Essential Facts

- Intradural lipomas without spinal dysraphism are only ~ 4% of spinal lipomas.
- Most patients have no neurologic symptoms at birth but may have cutaneous findings of a sacral dimple, skin tag, or hairy patch.
- If not diagnosed in infancy, sensory and motor deficits, orthopedic abnormalities including hammer toes and pes planus, and leg pain as well as urinary and fecal incontinence may develop.

◼ Other Imaging Findings

- Lipoma lying along the dorsal midline that is contained within the dural sac.
- No open spinal dysraphism, but there may be spina bifida at one or more levels.
- Most commonly lumbosacral.
- Low-lying conus (tethered cord).

✓ Pearls and ✗ Pitfalls

✓ Intradural spinal lipomas are the only type of spinal lipoma not always associated with a spinal dysraphism such as spina bifida or a lipomeningocele.

✗ Intradural lipomas are not isolated to the newborn period. They can occur in young adults where they are most commonly found in the upper thoracic and cervical spine.

Case 51

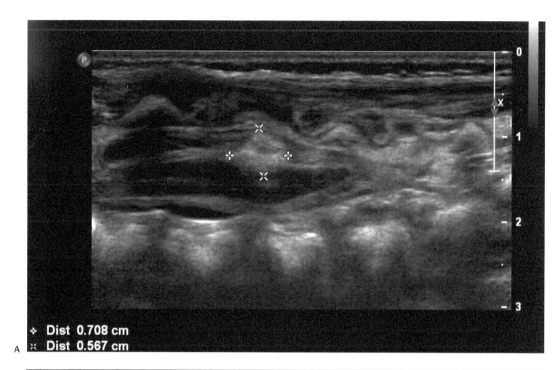

Dist 0.708 cm
Dist 0.567 cm

A

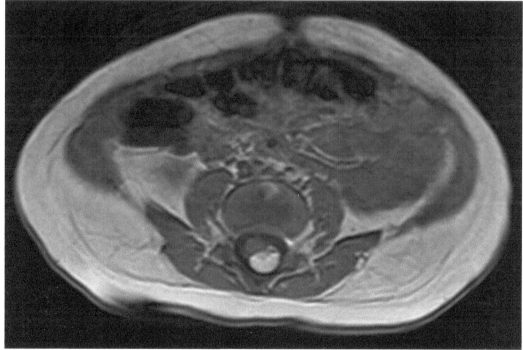

B

■ Clinical Presentation

A newborn with a sacral dimple.

■ Imaging Findings

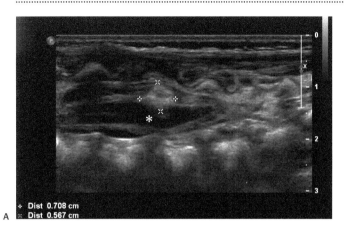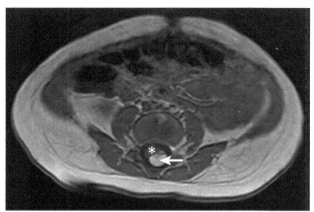

(A) Longitudinal ultrasound view of the lower lumbar spine. There is a subcentimeter echogenic mass (*calipers*) adjacent to the posterior surface of the spinal cord. It displaces the cord (*asterisk*) anteriorly. **(B)** Noncontrast axial T1 volumetric interpolated breath-hold examination MR image of the lumbar spine. There is an ovoid high signal intensity mass (*arrow*) in the left side of the spinal canal that displaces the cord (*asterisk*) to the right. It has the same signal intensity as fat but is not contiguous with the subcutaneous fat.

■ Differential Diagnosis

- ***Intradural lipoma:*** The T1 hyperintensity is consistent with fat. The fatty mass does not extend outside of the spinal canal or into the spine itself. No open spinal dysraphism is shown on these images.
- *Lipomyelomeningocele:* In lipomyelomeningocele, the lipoma is adjacent to a cleft in the spinal cord and extends into the central canal of the cord as well as into the spinal canal. The lipoma is continuous with the subcutaneous fat and is covered by intact skin.
- *Fibrolipoma of the filum terminale:* In this situation, the hyperintense T1 signal would be within the filum terminale instead of adjacent to the cord.

■ Essential Facts

- Intradural lipomas without spinal dysraphism are only ~ 4% of spinal lipomas.
- Most patients have no neurologic symptoms at birth but may have cutaneous findings of a sacral dimple, skin tag, or hairy patch.
- If not diagnosed in infancy, sensory and motor deficits, orthopedic abnormalities including hammer toes and pes planus, and leg pain as well as urinary and fecal incontinence may develop.

■ Other Imaging Findings

- Lipoma lying along the dorsal midline that is contained within the dural sac.
- No open spinal dysraphism, but there may be spina bifida at one or more levels.
- Most commonly lumbosacral.
- Low-lying conus (tethered cord).

✓ Pearls and ✗ Pitfalls

- ✓ Intradural spinal lipomas are the only type of spinal lipoma not always associated with a spinal dysraphism such as spina bifida or a lipomeningocele.
- ✗ Intradural lipomas are not isolated to the newborn period. They can occur in young adults where they are most commonly found in the upper thoracic and cervical spine.

Case 52

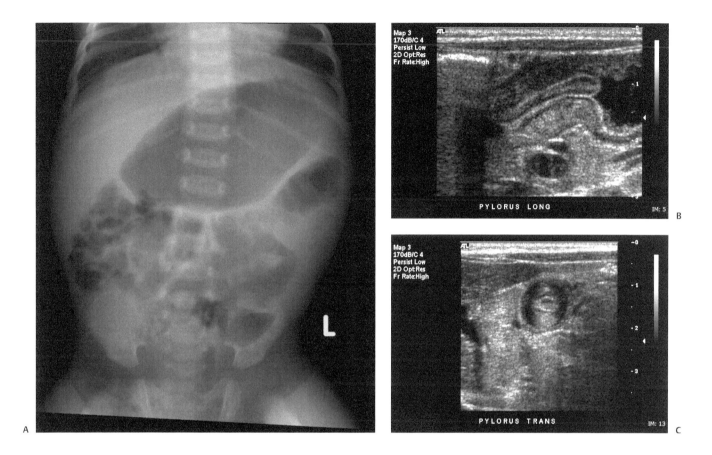

■ Clinical Presentation

A 5-week-old boy with persistent vomiting.

■ Imaging Findings

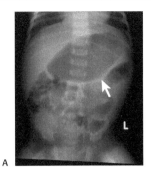 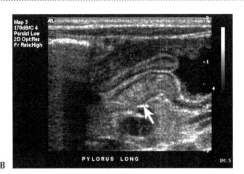 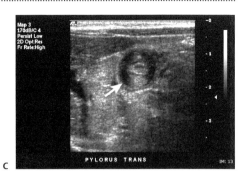

(A) Abdominal radiograph demonstrates a dilated stomach (*arrow*), with no dilation of the more distal bowel. **(B)** Longitudinal view of the pylorus demonstrates both elongation and thickening of the pyloric channel, which measures ~20 mm long (*arrow*). **(C)** Transverse view of the pylorus demonstrates circumferential thickening of the pyloric wall, which measures ~4 mm wide (*arrow*).

■ Differential Diagnosis

- **Hypertrophic pyloric stenosis:** Idiopathic thickening of the pyloric muscle causes gastric outlet obstruction associated with nonbilious projectile vomiting.
- *Pylorospasm:* During transient spasm, the pylorus can appear abnormally thickened and elongated. With observation over several minutes, however, spasm will resolve and the pylorus will be seen to relax, reducing the thickness of the muscle and opening up the pyloric channel.
- *Malrotation with midgut volvulus:* An important cause of vomiting in infants, but the vomitus in midgut volvulus is typically bilious, whereas in pyloric stenosis it is nonbilious.

■ Essential Facts

- Seen in infants between several weeks and several months of age.
- Male-to-female ratio is 5:1.
- Treated with pyloromyotomy.

■ Other Imaging Findings

- On barium upper gastrointestinal exam, there is "shouldering" of the gastric antrum, "tram-tracking" or severe narrowing of pyloric channel, and a "mushroom" sign of the duodenal bulb, all due to mass effect from the hypertrophied pyloric muscle.

✓ Pearls and ✗ Pitfalls

- ✓ Using ultrasound, watching the pylorus over several minutes helps to distinguish pylorospasm from hypertrophic pyloric stenosis.
- ✗ Lack of gastric distention on plain radiographs does not rule out the diagnosis of hypertrophic pyloric stenosis, because the stomach may be decompressed from vomiting.
- ✗ Imaging findings continue to resemble hypertrophic pyloric stenosis for a few weeks after pyloromyotomy.

Case 53

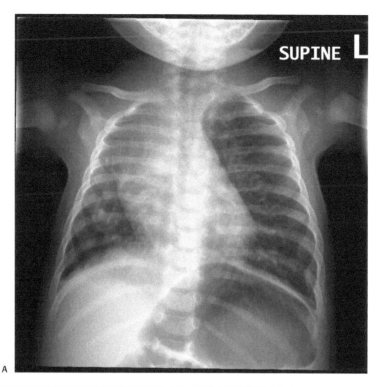

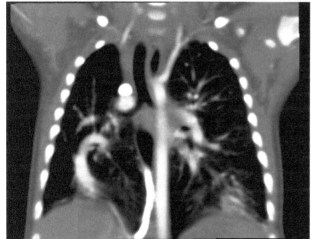

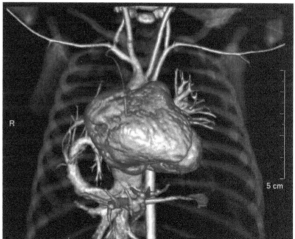

■ Clinical Presentation

A 2-month-old girl with respiratory distress.

■ Imaging Findings

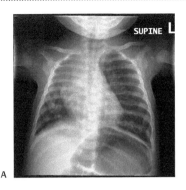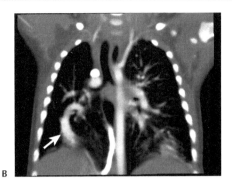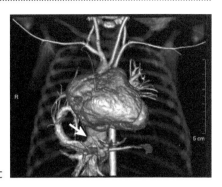

(A) Frontal chest radiograph demonstrates rightward shift of the heart and what appears to be an abnormal vessel coursing inferomedially from the right mid-lung. **(B)** Postcontrast coronal chest CT image better demonstrates the shape and course of the aberrant vessel (*arrow*). **(C)** Three-dimensional CT image in the coronal plane demonstrates that the aberrant pulmonary vein drains into the inferior vena cava (*arrow*).

■ Differential Diagnosis

- **Scimitar syndrome:** The classic features of scimitar syndrome include a hypoplastic right lung and anomalous pulmonary venous drainage, typically into the inferior vena cava, and systemic arterial supply of a portion of the right lung; the scimitar (Turkish sword)-shaped anomalous vessel is classic.
- *Pulmonary sequestration:* An extralobar pulmonary sequestration includes anomalous pulmonary venous drainage to the systemic circulation, but there should be an associated lower lobe mass, not seen in this case.
- *Pulmonary hypoplasia:* Either lung can be hypoplastic, but isolated hypoplasia should not demonstrate an aberrant pulmonary vein, as seen in this case.

■ Essential Facts

- Also known as congenital venolobar syndrome.
- An acyanotic form of congenital heart disease, which can be associated with congestive heart failure.
- Can be treated by embolization of the aberrant systemic arterial supply.

■ Other Imaging Findings

- Right pulmonary veins do not enter the right atrium.
- Dextroposition of the heart but not dextrocardia.
- Can be associated with shunt vascularity.

✓ Pearls and ✗ Pitfalls

✓ Can be an incidental finding in an asymptomatic older child or adult.
✗ Failure to embolize preoperatively can lead to intraoperative hemorrhage.

Case 54

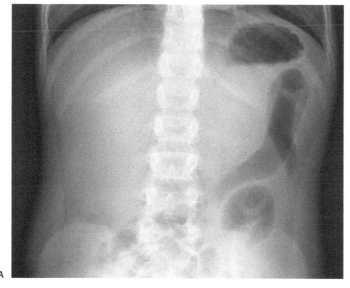

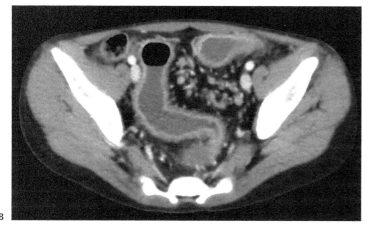

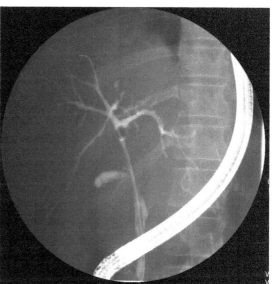

A 13-year-old boy with abdominal pain, bloody stools, and elevated markers for inflammation.

■ Imaging Findings

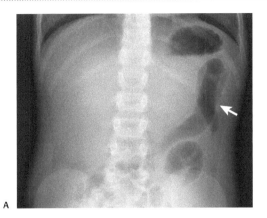

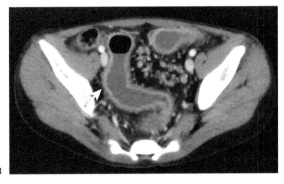

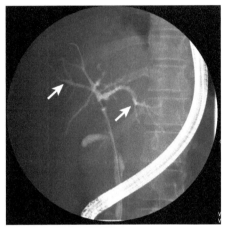

(A) Abdominal radiograph demonstrates a featureless appearance of the distal transverse and proximal descending colon (*arrow*). **(B)** Axial postcontrast CT image demonstrates wall thickening and increased mucosal enhancement of the sigmoid colon (*arrow*). **(C)** Endoscopic retrograde cholangiopancreatography demonstrates irregularity and a somewhat beaded appearance of the intrahepatic bile ducts (*arrows*), consistent with primary sclerosing cholangitis.

■ Differential Diagnosis

- ***Ulcerative colitis:*** The findings of a featureless colon with wall thickening and mucosal inflammation are consistent with ulcerative colitis; because a majority of patients with primary sclerosing cholangitis have ulcerative colitis, this makes this diagnosis especially likely.
- *Crohn disease:* Crohn disease often manifests with colonic disease and can be associated with primary sclerosing cholangitis, but there is no evidence of small bowel disease in this case and the bowel wall inflammation does not appear to be transmural.
- *Infectious colitis:* A variety of bacteria can cause colitis, but the small bowel is often involved as well, and such infections are not associated with primary sclerosing cholangitis.

■ Essential Facts

- Idiopathic inflammation of the colon that generally commences in the rectum and may advance proximally to involve the entire colon.

- Disease is continuous, as opposed to the "skip lesions" of Crohn disease.
- Colectomy is curative and eliminates the risk of colorectal cancer.

■ Other Imaging Findings

- Toxic megacolon, manifesting as colonic dilation and thumbprinting.
- Sclerosing cholangitis.
- Greatly increased risk of colorectal adenocarcinoma with longstanding disease.

✓ Pearls and ✗ Pitfalls

- ✓ Longstanding disease may result in rigid and narrowed "lead-pipe" colon.
- ✗ The diagnosis of ulcerative colitis should be considered in any patient diagnosed with primary sclerosing cholangitis.

Case 55

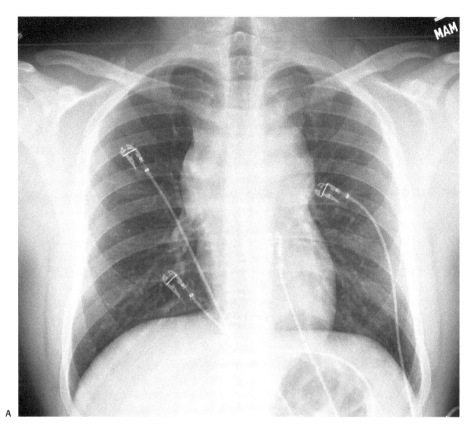

A

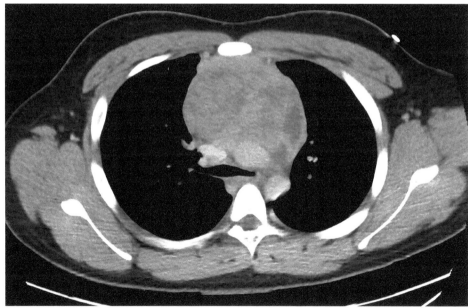

B

■ Clinical Presentation

A 16-year-old boy with chest pain.

■ Imaging Findings

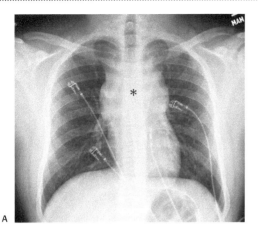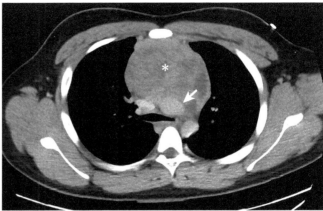

(A) Anteroposterior view X-ray of the chest shows abnormal widening of the mediastinum (*asterisk*). **(B)** Axial postcontrast CT image of the chest shows a heterogeneously enhancing soft tissue anterior mediastinal mass (*asterisk*) that displaces the great vessels (*arrow*) posteriorly.

■ Differential Diagnosis

- **Lymphoma:** A solid soft tissue mass in the anterior mediastinum is consistent with lymphoma.
- *Germ cell tumor:* Although this would also occur in the anterior mediastinum, the most common germ cell tumor in this age group is teratoma. Teratomas often contain fat and calcification, both of which are lacking in this tumor.
- *Thymus:* On chest X-ray, the normal thymus should not be visible in adolescents. On CT image, the thymus should not have mass effect on the vessels. The normal thymus should be minimal in a 16-year-old patient. Typically, by age 15 the thymus is smaller and more triangular and the margins are straight or concave.

■ Essential Facts

- Both Hodgkin and non-Hodgkin lymphoma can occur in children. Either type can cause anterior mediastinal masses; however, most anterior mediastinal masses in children are caused by Hodgkin lymphoma.

■ Other Imaging Findings

- Conglomerations of affected nodes rarely calcify before treatment but can calcify after treatment.
- Invasion of the pericardium is not uncommon and can lead to pericardial effusion.

✓ Pearls and ✗ Pitfalls

✓ Lymphoma is the most common cause of a mediastinal mass in children.
✓ When thinking of anterior mediastinal masses in children, consider the "4 Ts"—thymus, teratoma/germ cell tumors, thyroid, and "terrible lymphoma."
✗ In a child, a normal-appearing thymus can be confused with an anterior mediastinal mass.

Case 56

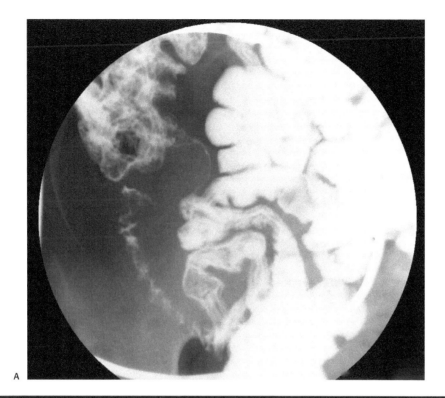

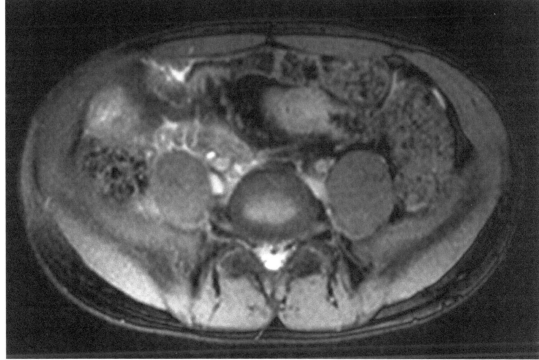

■ Clinical Presentation
....

A 15-year-old boy with diarrhea, fever, and leukocytosis.

■ Imaging Findings

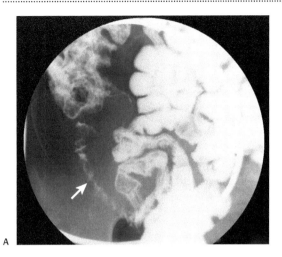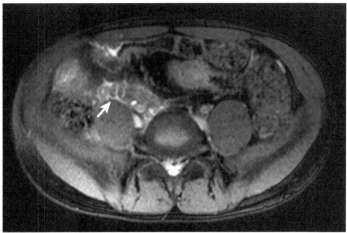

A   B

(A) Fluoroscopic image from a barium small bowel series demonstrates luminal narrowing and mural nodularity involving the terminal ileum (*arrow*). (B) Axial postcontrast T1-weighted image demonstrates bowel wall thickening and increased enhancement of the terminal ileum in the right lower quadrant (*arrow*).

■ Differential Diagnosis

- **Crohn disease:** The clinical history and imaging findings are typical for—although not diagnostic of—Crohn disease. Laboratory tests and biopsy are helpful in confirming the diagnosis.
- *Lymphoma:* As the largest lymphoid organ in the body, the gut is a relatively frequent site of involvement in lymphoma, which can present with wall thickening of the ileum, although perienteric inflammatory changes are not typical.
- *Infectious ileitis:* Infections of the ileum, such as *Yersinia*, can be associated with ileal bowel wall thickening, although the clinical course is generally more acute than in Crohn disease.

■ Other Imaging Findings

- Ulcers, sinus tracts, fistulas.
- Perianal disease.
- Bowel obstruction can be associated with strictures.

✓ Pearls and ✗ Pitfalls

✓ Increased risk of gallstones (due to disrupted enterohepatic circulation of bile salts) and nephrolithiasis (due to increased oxalate absorption).
✗ Beware increased risk of adenocarcinoma with longstanding disease.

■ Essential Facts

- Idiopathic inflammatory bowel disease.
- Transmural inflammation.
- Discontinuous involvement of any part of alimentary canal from mouth to anus.

Case 57

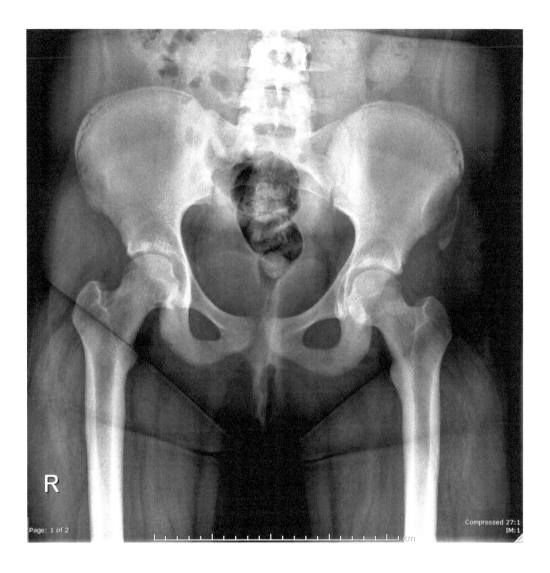

■ Clinical Presentation

A 12-year-old girl with abrupt onset of left hip pain.

■ Imaging Findings

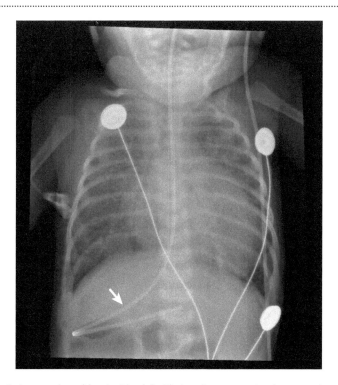

(A) Frontal chest radiograph demonstrates an enlarged heart with a left-sided cardiac apex and pulmonary edema, as well as a nasogastric tube that extends into the right upper quadrant, indicating a right-sided stomach (*arrow*).

■ Differential Diagnosis

- **Heterotaxy:** The contralateral position of cardiac apex and stomach is indicative of heterotaxy.
- *Situs inversus:* The stomach is right sided in situs inversus, but in this condition, the cardiac apex should also be on the right side.
- *Perforation of the esophagus:* A nasogastric tube can perforate the esophagus and extend into an atypical position, although associated findings such as pneumomediastinum, plural effusion, and possibly pneumoperitoneum should also be present.

■ Essential Facts

- Cardiac apex and stomach located on opposite sides.
- Two major types: Asplenia ("double right sidedness") and polysplenia ("double left sidedness").

- Asplenia seen in males who present early with severe cyanotic congenital heart disease.
- Polysplenia associated with less severe heart disease; often presents later.

■ Other Imaging Findings

- Asplenia—aorta and IVC on same side, bilateral tri-lobed lungs, anomalous pulmonary venous connection.
- Polysplenia—multiple spleens, azygous continuation of inferior vena cava, bilobed lungs.
- Intestinal malrotation.

✓ Pearls and ✗ Pitfalls

✓ Anatomy can be complex, requiring a step-by-step approach.
✗ Mortality higher in asplenia than in polysplenia.

Case 60

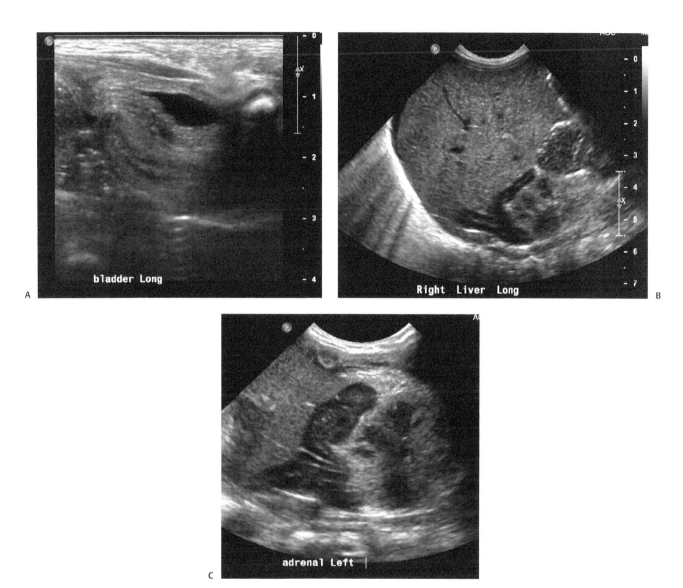

A

B

C

■ Clinical Presentation

A newborn with ambiguous genitalia.

▦ Imaging Findings

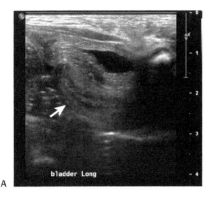 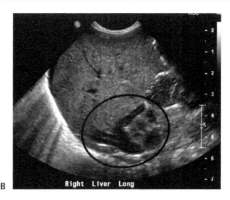 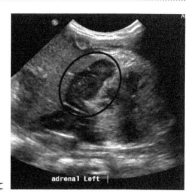

(A) Longitudinal grayscale ultrasound view of the pelvis. Posterior to the bladder, there is a uterus (*arrow*). **(B)** Longitudinal grayscale ultrasound view of the right liver gland. The right adrenal gland (*circle*) is prominent. The width of the limb is 6 mm and the length of the limb is 27 mm. **(C)** Longitudinal grayscale ultrasound view of the left adrenal gland. There is a cerebriform or coiled appearance of the left adrenal gland (*circle*).

▦ Differential Diagnosis

- ***Congenital adrenal hyperplasia (CAH):*** Enlarged, cerebriform adrenal glands in an infant with ambiguous genitalia and a uterus is consistent with CAH.
- *Normal newborn adrenal gland:* Although normal newborn adrenal glands can often be seen on ultrasound images, they should not be this large or cerebriform in appearance.
- *Partial androgen insensitivity:* Although this can present with ambiguous genitalia, it should not significantly impair female genitalia, only male. Because this patient has a uterus, she should not be affected.

▦ Essential Facts

- CAH is the most common cause of ambiguous genitalia.
- CAH manifests as various degrees of virilization in girls and precocious puberty in boys.
- Most cases are secondary to 21-hydroxylase deficiency causing an elevated level of 17-hydroxyprogesterone.

▦ Other Imaging Findings

- Bilateral adrenal glands with a single limb > 2 cm long and 4 mm wide and normal corticomedullary differentiation is suggestive of CAH.
- The adrenal gland may be lobulated and have a stippled echogenicity.
- Cerebriform or coiled appearance of the adrenal gland is specific for CAH.

- Females with CAH have a normal-appearing uterus and ovaries.
- Males with CAH may have testicular adrenal rest tumors that most commonly appear as bilateral spikelike intratesticular masses surrounding the mediastinal testes. If they are < 2 cm in size, they are typically hypoechoic; they are hyperechoic if > 2 cm. They are hypo- or avascular without distortion of vessels. Larger lesions may not be confined to the mediastinum. Lesions can even be seen in the epididymis or, if small, may be unilateral.
- Ovarian adrenal rest tumors can be seen as hypoechoic nodules on ultrasound.

✓ Pearls and ✗ Pitfalls

- ✓ Ambiguous genitalia with ultrasound findings of a uterus and enlarged adrenal glands is almost pathognomonic for CAH.
- ✓ The presence of polycystic ovaries is increased in women with CAH.
- ✓ In adults with CAH, adrenal nodules are common and often correlate with hormonal control status.
- ✗ The presence of normal-appearing adrenal glands does not rule out the diagnosis of CAH.

Case 61

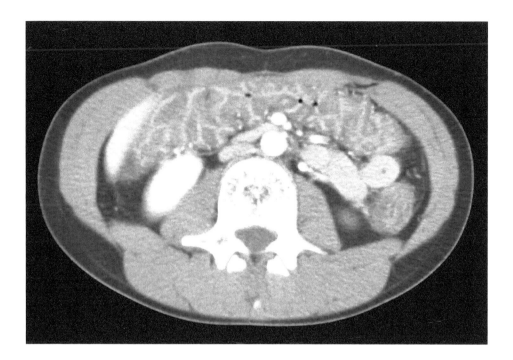

■ Clinical Presentation

A 13-year-old boy presents with bloody diarrhea 1 week after completing a course of antibiotics.

■ Imaging Findings

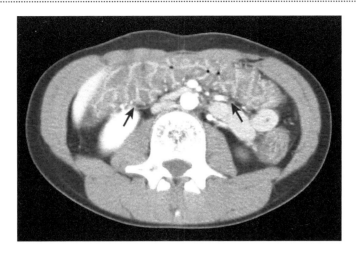

(A) An axial postcontrast CT image demonstrates marked wall thickening, edema, and mucosal enhancement involving the transverse (*arrows*) and proximal descending colon.

■ Differential Diagnosis

- ***Pseudomembranous colitis:*** The history of antibiotic use and diarrhea are typical, as is the nodular, edematous wall thickening and mucosal enhancement involving all visualized portions of the colon.
- *Ulcerative colitis:* Ulcerative colitis often involves the entire colon, but the degree of wall thickening in this case is greater than usually seen with ulcerative colitis, and the history of recent antibiotic use is not typical.
- *Neutropenic colitis:* Neutropenic colitis can cause similar bowel wall thickening and edema, but it often involves only the right side of the colon, and in this case, the patient has no history of neutropenia.

■ Essential Facts

- Colitis due to overgrowth of *Clostridium difficile* associated with prior antibiotic therapy.
- Diagnosis made from stool samples but treatment often initiated based on history and imaging findings.
- In severe cases, colectomy may be required.

■ Other Imaging Findings

- Thumbprinting due to thickened haustral folds may be visible on abdominal radiographs.
- "Accordion sign" describes alternating bands of bright luminal contrast and darker thickened folds.
- Bowel wall thickening is often much greater than the degree of pericolonic inflammation.

✓ Pearls and ✕ Pitfalls

- ✓ Fecal transplants are playing a growing role in therapy.
- ✕ Contrast enema and endoscopy should generally be avoided due to risk of perforation.

Case 62

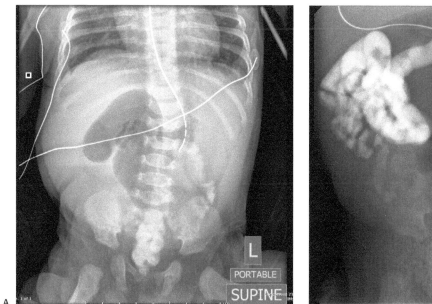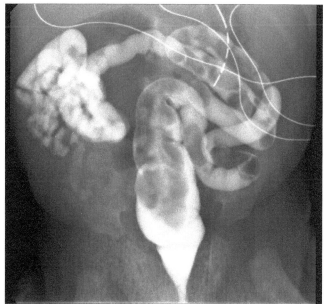

Clinical Presentation

A 2-day-old with failure to pass meconium. Prior enema at outside hospital was not diagnostic.

■ Imaging Findings

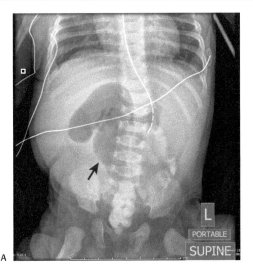
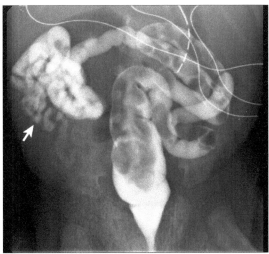

(A) Abdominal radiograph demonstrates marked dilation of several segments of bowel in the upper abdomen (*arrow*), suggestive of a high-grade bowel obstruction. (B) Abdominal radiograph from a contrast enema demonstrates a normal caliber rectum, but the remainder of the colon is small. There is reflux of contrast into the ileum, which contains very little meconium (*arrow*). Contrast could not be refluxed into the dilated segments of small bowel.

■ Differential Diagnosis

- *Ileal atresia:* The findings of a microcolon with abrupt interruption of contrast reflux through nondilated ileum is consistent with ileal atresia.
- *Meconium plug syndrome:* In meconium plug syndrome, the colon distal to the splenic flexure is usually small in caliber, whereas the colon proximal to the splenic flexure is usually dilated. In this case, there is no change in caliber at or near the splenic flexure.
- *Meconium ileus:* The appearance of the colon is consistent with meconium ileus, although the segments of ileum into which contrast was refluxed do not exhibit multiple filling defects—the inspissated meconium that should be present in meconium ileus.

■ Essential Facts

- Ileal atresia typically presents in the first day or two of life with abdominal distention and failure to pass meconium.
- The pathophysiology of ileal atresia is thought to be an in utero vascular accident, in part because it is typically accompanied by a defect in the adjacent small bowel mesentery.

- On plain radiographs, ileal atresia can appear very similar to a number of other causes of neonatal bowel obstruction, including meconium plug syndrome, meconium ileus, and Hirschsprung disease. The contrast enema is the key to diagnosis.
- Surgical resection of the atretic segment is required.

■ Other Imaging Findings

- The more distal the point of bowel obstruction, the more the dilated bowel is likely to be apparent on abdominal radiography.
- When there is a congenital bowel obstruction at the level of the ileum, contrast enema is likely to reveal a microcolon.

✓ Pearls and ✗ Pitfalls

- ✓ Low-osmolar and iso-osmolar contrast agents help to prevent large shifts of fluid into the bowel lumen.
- ✓ At surgery, some patients have multiple points of atresia.
- ✗ Barium is not used for neonatal contrast enemas, partly because of the danger of barium peritonitis in case of a perforation, and also because it may interfere with the passage of meconium.

Case 63

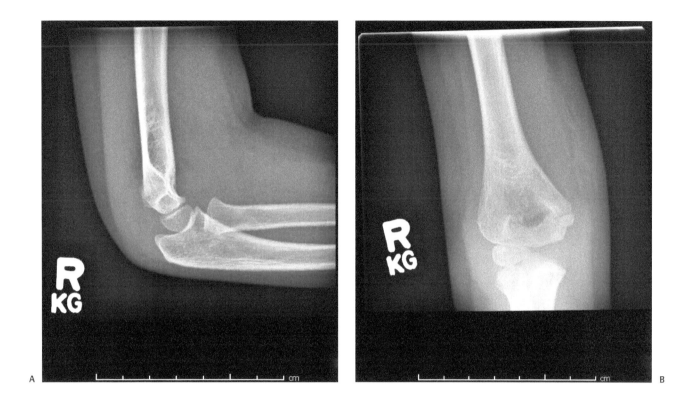

A   B

■ Clinical Presentation

A 6-year-old girl with elbow pain after a fall.

▣ Imaging Findings

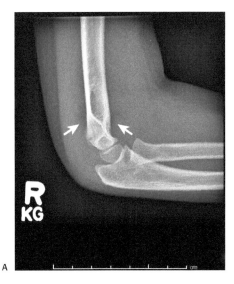 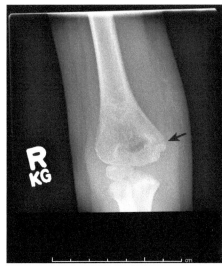

(A) Lateral radiography of the elbow demonstrates prominent anterior and posterior fat pads (*arrows*), indicating an elbow joint effusion but no definite fracture. **(B)** Frontal elbow radiograph demonstrates a transverse linear lucency extending across the medial aspect of the distal humerus (*arrow*).

▣ Differential Diagnosis

- ***Supracondylar fracture:*** The combination of pain after trauma, prominent fat pads, and transverse lucency is indicative of a nondisplaced (type 1) supracondylar fracture.
- *Arthritis:* An inflammatory or infectious arthritis of the elbow can cause a joint effusion and elevation of the anterior and posterior fat pads, but such conditions should not be associated with the lucency on the frontal view.
- *Medial condyle fracture:* A fracture isolated to the medial condyle of the elbow is relatively rare and would not be positioned in this plane.

▣ Essential Facts

- Most common pediatric elbow fracture (radial fractures more common in adults).
- Often associated with posterior displacement of the distal fragment.
- No visible fracture line in a quarter of patients, in whom follow-up radiographs obtained a week later typically demonstrate the fracture.

▣ Other Imaging Findings

- With posterior displacement/angulation of the distal fragment, the anterior humeral line will not intersect the middle third of the capitellum.
- CT or MRI can confirm radiographically occult fracture.
- Displaced fracture can result in neurovascular injury.

✓ Pearls and ✗ Pitfalls

- ✓ Most supracondylar fractures result from extension injuries.
- ✗ Check for associated olecranon and medial epicondyle fractures.

Case 64

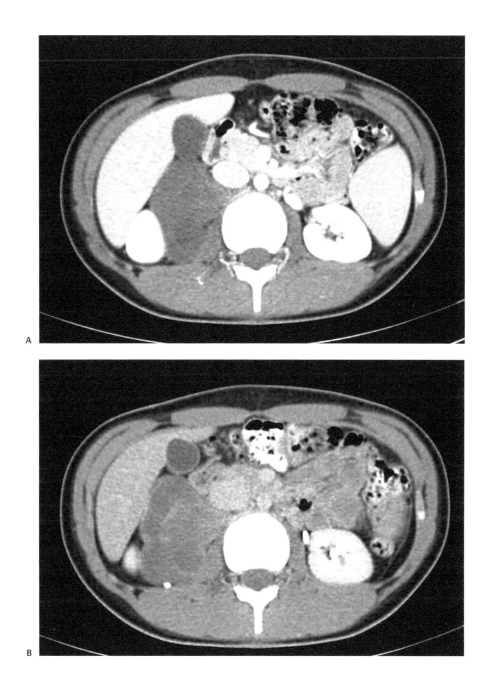

■ Clinical Presentation

A 14-year-old girl with abdominal pain.

■ Imaging Findings

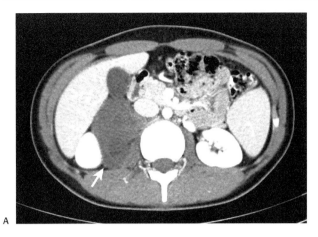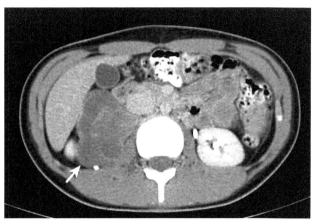

A   B

(A) Postcontrast axial abdominal CT image obtained in the arterial phase demonstrates a multilobular cystic mass in the right upper quadrant (*arrow*), filling in the space between the right kidney and inferior vena cava. It demonstrates minimal peripheral enhancement. **(B)** Postcontrast axial CT scan at the same level, obtained during the urographic phase (note contrast in the left renal collecting system and ureter) demonstrates increased peripheral enhancement of the lesion but minimal or no central enhancement (*arrow*).

■ Differential Diagnosis

- ***Venolymphatic malformation:*** The multilobular, multiseptated appearance of the lesion combined with its delayed and peripheral enhancement is most consistent with a venolymphatic malformation.
- *Enteric duplication cyst:* Enteric duplication cysts are generally round or ovoid and have a well-defined, enhancing wall.
- *Mesenteric cyst:* These lesions may have a multiseptated appearance, but they are typically found along the mesenteric border of the bowel.

■ Essential Facts

- Slow-flow lesion consisting of dilated venous and lymphatic channels that are often filled with proteinaceous fluid.
- Thought to be congenital.
- May enlarge over time, and enlargement can be abrupt in hemorrhage and infection.
- Can be treated with sclerotherapy.

■ Other Imaging Findings

- Comprised of unenhancing or poorly enhancing cysts.
- May cross normal anatomic boundaries, insinuating themselves between normal anatomic structures.
- With hemorrhage, may demonstrate fluid–fluid levels.

✓ Pearls and ✗ Pitfalls

- ✓ Microcystic lesions may have a more solid appearance.
- ✗ Can be difficult to differentiate from other vascular lesions, particularly on ultrasound.

Case 65

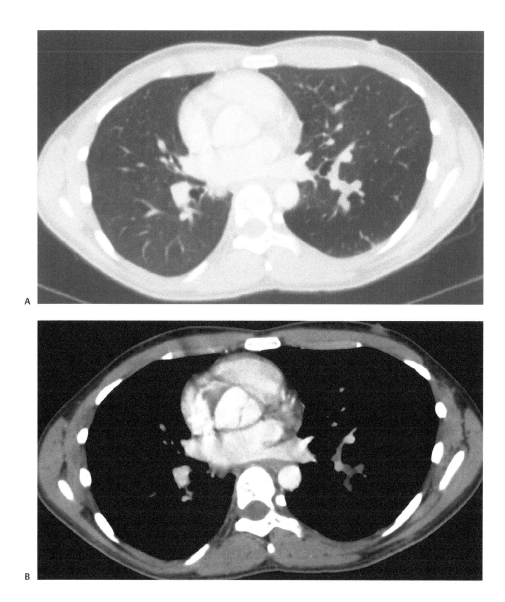

A 16-year-old boy with history of pneumonia.

▦ Imaging Findings

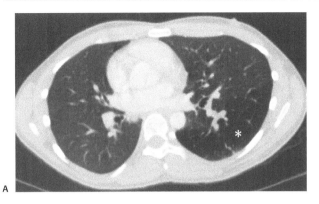
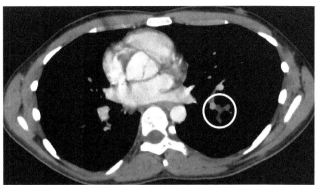

(A) Axial CT image of the chest, lung windows. In the left lower lobe, there is air trapping (*asterisk*). **(B)** Axial CT image of the chest, soft tissue windows. There is a tubular, nonenhancing branching structure (*circle*) in the same area as the air trapping.

▦ Differential Diagnosis

- ***Congenital bronchial atresia:*** The athletic bronchi with distal impacted mucus (mucocele or bronchocele) with surrounding air trapping is consistent with bronchial atresia.
- *Allergic bronchopulmonary aspergillosis (ABPA):* This usually occurs in patients with longstanding asthma or cystic fibrosis. The CT usually demonstrates saccular bronchiectasis. The impacted mucus may be calcified (high density).
- *Pulmonary AVM:* Although AVM would be tubular in appearance, it should enhance with the other vessels.

▦ Essential Facts

- Congenital bronchial atresia results from interruption of a bronchus with distal mucus impaction and hyperexpansion of the obstructed segment.
- Usually discovered incidentally. If symptomatic, may cause shortness of breath; cough; or, less likely, infection.

▦ Other Imaging Findings

- Chest X-ray may show the bronchocele as a tubular, round, ovoid, or branching density.
- Inspiration and expiration may help to confirm that the affected lung is hyperinflated.

✓ Pearls and ✗ Pitfalls

- ✓ The configuration of the impacted mucus has been referred to as the "finger-in-glove sign" due to the branching. It can also appear as the letter V or Y depending on the number of bronchi involved.
- ✗ CT findings are typical; however, resection may be done to rule out the rare possibility of a small malignancy as the cause of obstruction.
- ✗ Bronchoceles can be seen in other pathologies such as cystic fibrosis, allergic bronchopulmonary aspergillosis, and impacted foreign body.

Case 66

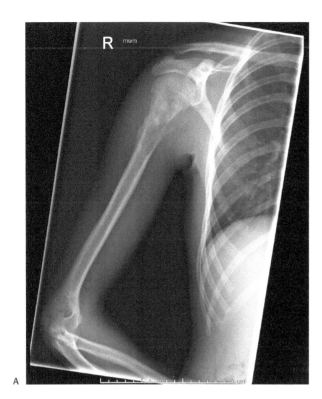

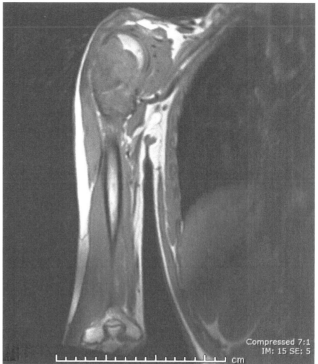

■ Clinical Presentation

A 16-year-old boy with right arm pain.

■ Imaging Findings

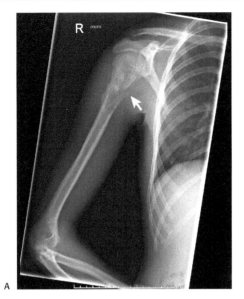 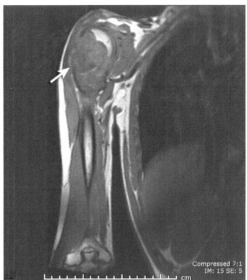

(A) Frontal humerus radiograph demonstrates a predominately lytic lesion in the proximal humerus with Codman triangle (*arrow*), suggesting an aggressive lesion. **(B)** Coronal T1-weighted MR image demonstrates a hypointense mass extending from the metaphysis both down into the diaphysis and up into the epiphysis and extending beyond the expected margins of the bone (*arrow*).

■ Differential Diagnosis

- ***Osteosarcoma:*** The finding of a lytic, aggressive metaphyseal mass that extends into the epiphysis is typical of an osteosarcoma.
- *Ewing sarcoma:* Ewing sarcomas are more likely to arise in the diaphysis of long bones and typically demonstrate no osteoid production.
- *Aneurysmal bone cyst:* Aneurysmal bone cysts are lytic, often expansile lesions, but they should not be associated with a soft tissue mass or aggressive features such as Codman triangle.

■ Essential Facts

- Most common primary bone malignancy in pediatric patients.
- Most commonly arises in the metaphysis of a long bone.
- Aggressive features: poorly defined zone of transition, sunburst or Codman triangle pattern of periosteal reaction.
- Often associated with osteoid formation.

■ Other Imaging Findings

- Intense radiotracer uptake on bone scan, which can be used for staging.
- Chest CT to assess for pulmonary metastases.
- MRI to assess extent of tumor, joint involvement, relationship to nerves and blood vessels.
- MRI also used to assess treatment response prior to resection.

✓ Pearls and ✓ Pitfalls

- ✓ Plain radiograph best to determine lesion type, MRI best for treatment planning.
- ✗ On MR image, presence of fluid–fluid levels does not prove lesion is an aneurysmal bone cyst, because telangiectatic osteosarcomas can have a similar appearance.

Case 67

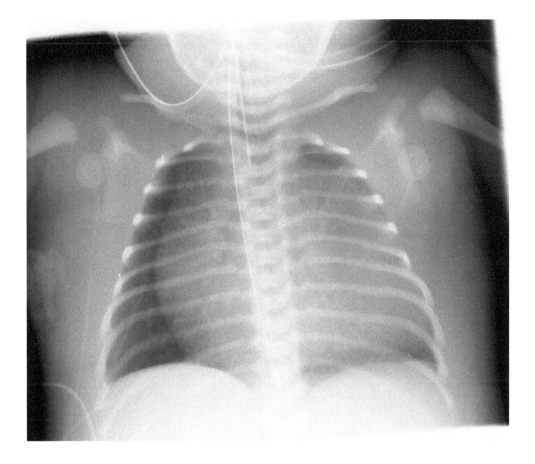

A 1-day-old girl who is cyanotic, with respiratory distress requiring mechanical ventilation.

■ Imaging Findings

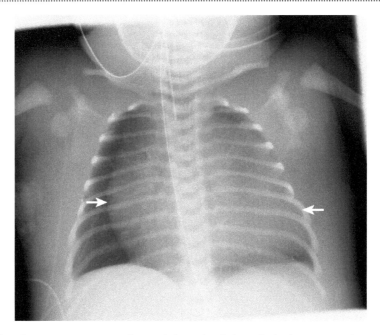

(A) Frontal radiograph of the chest demonstrates massive cardiomegaly (*arrows*) with diminished pulmonary vascularity.

■ Differential Diagnosis

- **Ebstein anomaly:** Ebstein anomaly is a form of cyanotic congenital heart disease that is classically associated with a massive, box-shaped heart and diminished pulmonary vascularity.
- *Pericardial effusion:* A large pericardial effusion can cause impressive enlargement of the cardiac shadow, although it should not cause cyanosis.
- *Pulmonary atresia with intact ventricular septum:* With severe tricuspid regurgitation, this lesion can also cause cyanosis and severe cardiomegaly and typically requires echocardiography for differentiation.

■ Essential Facts

- Displacement of the tricuspid valve leaflets downward into the right ventricle.
- "Atrialization" of a portion of the right ventricle.
- Enlargement of the right atrium, often massive.
- Possible association with maternal lithium use.

■ Other Imaging Findings

- Heart can be nearly normal in size in neonate, gradually enlarging over time.
- Echocardiography and MR image show tricuspid regurgitation.
- Often associated with atrial septal defect.

✓ Pearls and ✗ Pitfalls

- ✓ Definitive repair involves tricuspid valve replacement.
- ✗ Patients may develop arrhythmias that can be associated with sudden death.

Case 68

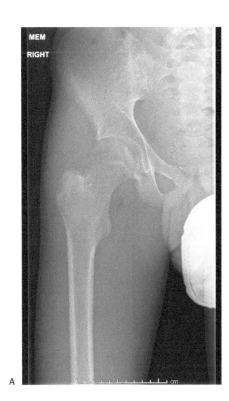

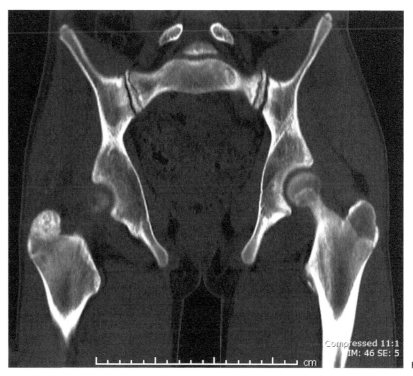

■ Clinical Presentation

A 15-year-old boy with right hip pain.

■ Imaging Findings

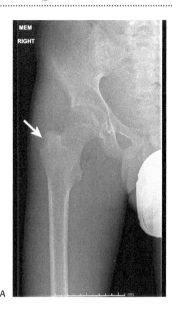
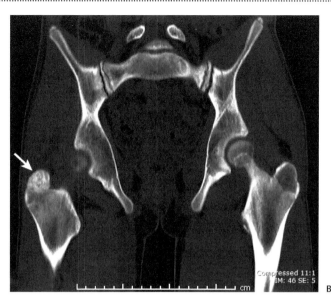

(A) A frontal radiograph of the right hip demonstrates a lytic lesion in the right femoral greater trochanter that contains "ring and arc"-like calcifications (*arrow*).
(B) Coronal CT image better demonstrates the geographic borders of the lesion as well as the chondroid pattern of internal calcification (*arrow*).

■ Differential Diagnosis

- **Chondroblastoma:** The location, an epiphysis or epiphyseal equivalent (as in this case); the nonaggressive appearance; and the particular pattern of calcification are all typical of chondroblastoma.
- *Langerhans cell histiocytosis:* Langerhans cell histiocytosis could present in the greater trochanter, but the lesion is usually more purely lytic without internal calcifications, and cortical destruction is a frequent feature.
- *Osteomyelitis:* Osteomyelitis can occur in the greater trochanter, but more aggressive features such as periosteal reaction would typically be present.

■ Essential Facts

- Benign tumor of immature cartilage cells.
- Located in an epiphysis or epiphyseal equivalent.
- May extend into the metaphysis.

■ Other Imaging Findings

- Heterogeneous on MR image.
- A third of patients develop a secondary aneurysmal bone cyst.
- Treated with curettage and bone grafting.

✓ Pearls and ✗ Pitfalls

✓ Most common in the second decade of life.
✗ Many patients have been experiencing symptoms for >1 year at the time of diagnosis.

Case 69

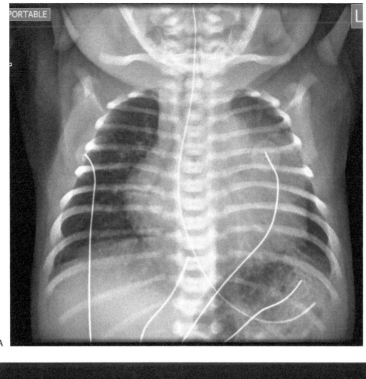

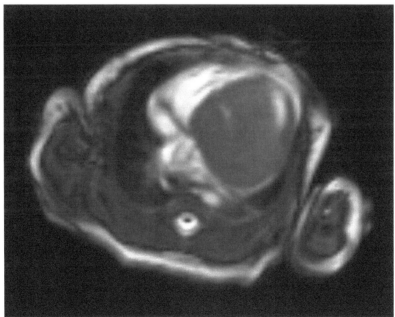

■ Clinical Presentation

A 2-day-old girl with respiratory distress.

■ Imaging Findings

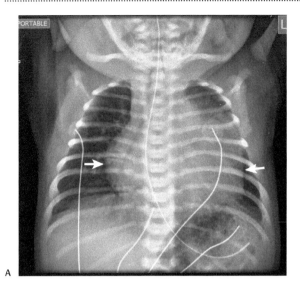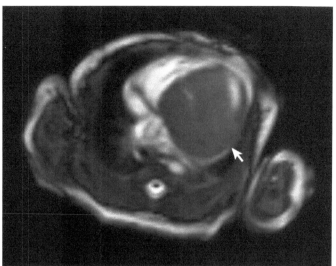

(A) Frontal chest radiograph demonstrates cardiomegaly (*arrows*) and mild central pulmonary edema. **(B)** Axial T1-weighted MR image demonstrates a large isointense mass occupying much of the left ventricle (*arrow*).

■ Differential Diagnosis

- **Cardiac rhabdomyoma:** Cardiac rhabdomyomas can present as small or large masses that often arise from the interventricular septum and typically appear isointense on T1-weighted MR images.
- *Cardiac fibroma:* One of the most common benign congenital cardiac masses, fibromas can also appear isointense on MR image.
- *Myxoma:* Cardiac myxomas can present as large masses in cardiac chambers, but they are generally seen in older adults and tend to arise in the left atrium.

■ Essential Facts

- Hamartoma.
- Associated with tuberous sclerosis.
- Size and location of mass determine symptoms; many small masses are asymptomatic.
- Generally resolve spontaneously over several years.

■ Other Imaging Findings

- Renal angiomyolipomas.
- Subependymal nodules.
- Giant cell astrocytoma.
- Lymphangioleiomyomatosis.

✓ Pearls and ✗ Pitfalls

✓ Most common congenital cardiac tumor.
✗ Lesions are often multiple.

Case 70

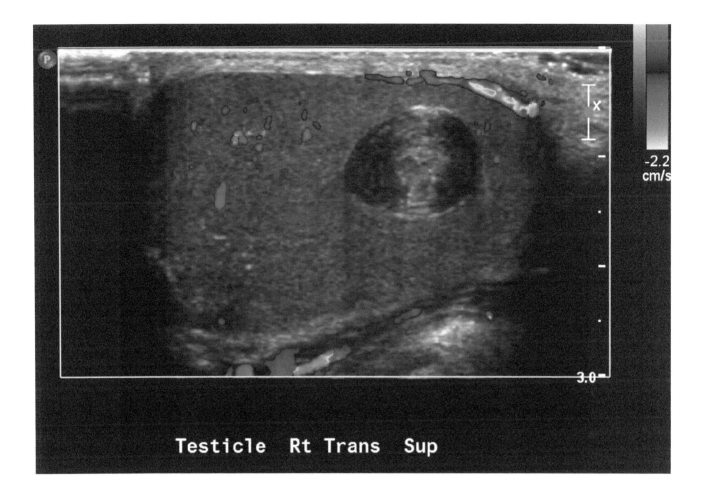

Testicle Rt Trans Sup

■ Clinical Presentation

A 15-year-old boy with a painless testicular mass.

■ Imaging Findings

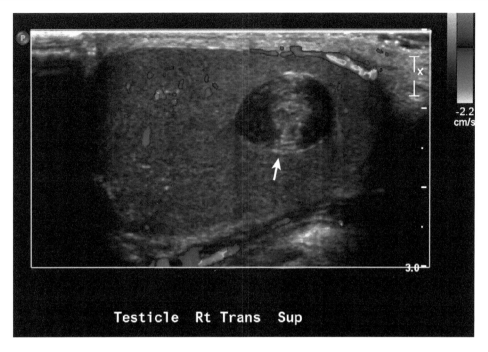

(A) Transverse color Doppler ultrasound image of the right testicle. There is a well-defined mass with a lamellated appearance of alternating hyper- and hypoechoic rings (*arrow*). There is no internal blood flow.

■ Differential Diagnosis

- **Epidermoid:** The classic onion skin or whorled appearance without internal blood flow is typical of an epidermoid.
- *Nonseminomatous germ cell tumor (NSGCT):* Although a malignant tumor cannot be ruled out by imaging alone, NSGCT tends to be more heterogeneous with internal blood flow.
- *Abscess:* Although abscesses can be round, they typically have irregular borders and heterogeneous centers surrounded by a rim of hypervascularity. In addition, they usually are not painless.

■ Essential Facts

- Epidermoids have no malignant potential. Complete resection of the tumor is curative.
- They are composed of alternating layers of keratinous debris lined with keratinizing squamous epithelium.

■ Other Imaging Findings

- Epidermoids can have a rim of hypoechogenicity with central hyperechogenicity resembling a target sign.
- On MR image, they tend to be well defined and may show alternating rings of high and low signal on both T1- and T2-weighted images. They typically show no contrast enhancement.

✓ Pearls and ✗ Pitfalls

- ✓ Most common benign tumor in prepubertal patients is an epidermoid.
- ✓ A high index of suspicion must be maintained for a malignant lesion because they are 50 times more common than testicular epidermoids in young men.
- ✗ Although the lamellated appearance is characteristic of epidermoids, it is not pathognomonic. The mass should be evaluated for any irregular borders, which suggest a malignant lesion.

Case 71

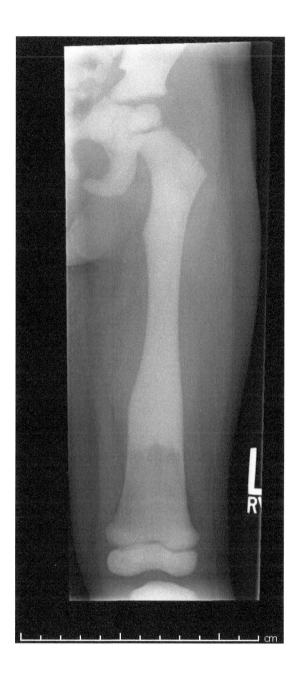

■ Clinical Presentation

A 3-year-old girl with leg pain.

■ Imaging Findings

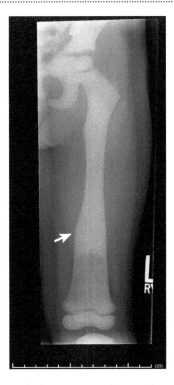

(A) Frontal radiograph of the left femur demonstrates unusually dense-appearing bones with an "Erlenmeyer flask" deformity of the distal femur (*arrow*).

■ Differential Diagnosis

- **Osteopetrosis:** The dramatically increased density and "Erlenmeyer flask" deformity are indicative of osteopetrosis.
- *Fibrous dysplasia:* Fibrous dysplasia can cause a sclerotic, expansile appearance, but when it affects the femur, it often causes bowing, not found in this case. Moreover, in this case, the contralateral femur had an identical appearance, which would be unusual for fibrous dysplasia.
- *Renal osteodystrophy:* Patients with chronic renal failure can develop diffuse bony sclerosis, although it would not be associated with an "Erlenmeyer flask" deformity, and there is no history of renal failure in this case.

■ Essential Facts

- A disorder of osteoclast function that prevents bone remodeling and results in narrowing of the medullary cavity.
- Bones are dense but brittle, with increased risk of fracture.
- Can be associated with anemia and cranial nerve palsies.

■ Other Imaging Findings

- Vertebral end plates are often sclerotic.
- Pelvic bones often exhibit a "bone within bone" appearance.
- Skull base often appears dense.

✓ Pearls and ✗ Pitfalls

- ✓ Bone marrow transplantation can be curative.
- ✗ Patients often present with pathologic fractures.

Case 72

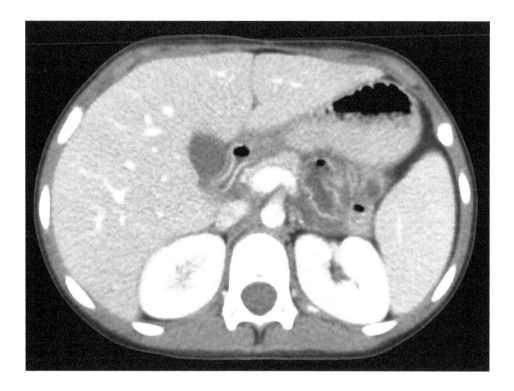

A 4-year-old boy presents with bilious emesis and palpable purpura.

■ Imaging Findings

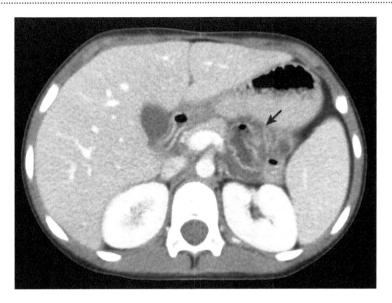

(A) Axial postcontrast CT image of the abdomen demonstrates increased mucosal enhancement and intramural edema of the proximal jejunum (*arrow*).

■ Differential Diagnosis

- ***Henoch–Schönlein purpura:*** Bowel wall inflammation and edema are a common manifestation of Henoch–Schönlein purpura, which as the name implies, is commonly characterized by purpuric skin lesions.
- *Infectious enteritis:* Infectious enteritis can also be associated with vomiting and increased mucosal enhancement and bowel wall edema, although it is not typically associated with a skin rash.
- *Child abuse:* Child abuse can present with skin lesions (burns and bruising) and bowel injury resembling these imaging finding, but palpable purpura is not a feature of child abuse.

■ Essential Facts

- Idiopathic immune-complex deposition vasculitis associated with a triad of purpuric rash on legs, abdominal pain, and joint symptoms.
- Occurs most commonly in the mid–first decade of life.
- Multiorgan system disease that can involve the urinary and musculoskeletal systems.
- No therapy proven to shorten disease course.

■ Other Imaging Findings

- Often associated with scrotal inflammation, manifesting as scrotal wall thickening.
- Half of patients have renal involvement, with enlargement and increased echogenicity.
- Radiographs of joints typically show only soft tissue swelling.

✓ Pearls and ✗ Pitfalls

- ✓ Gastrointestinal symptoms are most common at presentation.
- ✓ Increases risk of enteroenteric intussusception.
- ✗ Disease can recur months after initial presentation.

Case 73

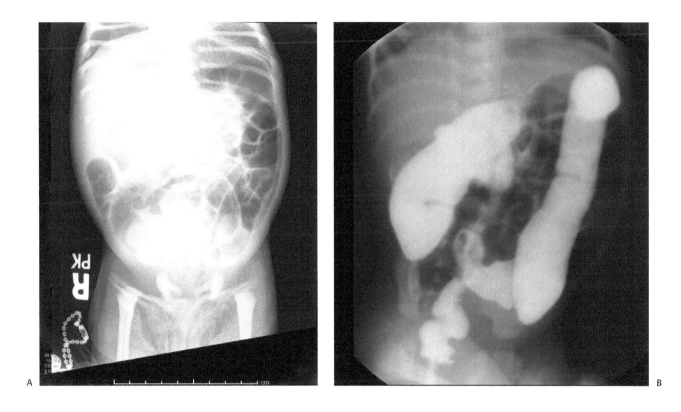

A

B

■ Clinical Presentation

A 2-day-old with bilious vomiting and failure to pass meconium.

■ Imaging Findings

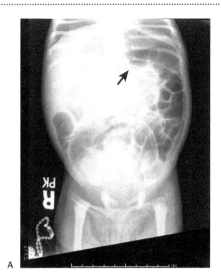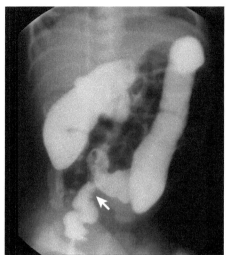

(A) Abdominal radiograph demonstrates dilated bowel filling the entire abdomen, strongly suggestive of a distal bowel obstruction. An orogastric tube tip is in the stomach (*arrow*). **(B)** Abdominal radiograph from a contrast enema demonstrates a relatively small-caliber rectum (*arrow*), as compared to the sigmoid colon and the bowel proximal to it.

■ Differential Diagnosis

- **Hirschsprung disease:** The finding of a rectosigmoid caliber ratio that is < 1, meaning that the rectum is smaller in caliber than the sigmoid colon, is strongly suggestive of Hirschsprung disease.
- *Meconium plug syndrome:* Presents with a distal bowel obstruction, but on contrast enema the transition point between nondilated distal colon and dilated proximal colon is typically more proximal than in this case, at the level of the splenic flexure.
- *Ileal atresia:* Again, presents with a distal bowel obstruction, but on contrast enema the entire colon is small, not just the rectum and distal sigmoid colon as in this case.

■ Essential Facts

- Due to embryonic interruption of caudal migration of neural crest cells, with the result that the distal colon lacks normal innervation and remains contracted, causing a functional bowel obstruction.
- Diagnosis is established by suction biopsy, which shows absence of ganglion cells in the affected distal segment of bowel.
- Milder cases may present later in infancy.

■ Other Imaging Findings

- Spasm of the affected segment of bowel is associated with an irregular mucosal contour on contrast enema.
- Evacuation of contrast after enema is often delayed in patients with Hirschsprung disease.
- Surgical treatment involves resection of the aganglionic segment with pull-through of normal bowel and anastomosis with the anus.

✓ Pearls and ✗ Pitfalls

- ✓ Early filling lateral view of the rectum can be very helpful in assessing the rectosigmoid ratio and detecting a transition zone.
- ✓ Once a point of transition in colonic caliber is encountered, there is no need to continue refluxing contrast material proximally.
- ✗ Hirschsprung disease can affect the entire colon; in this case, no point of transition in caliber will be encountered.
- ✗ A normal contrast enema does not exclude Hirschsprung disease, and if clinical suspicion is high, suction biopsy should be performed in any case.

Case 74

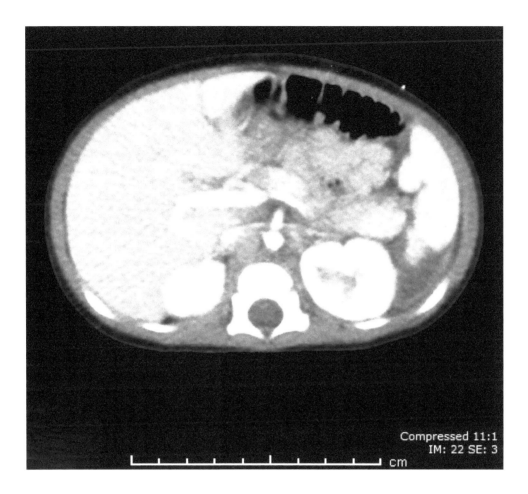

■ Clinical Presentation

A child struck by a motor vehicle.

■ Imaging Findings

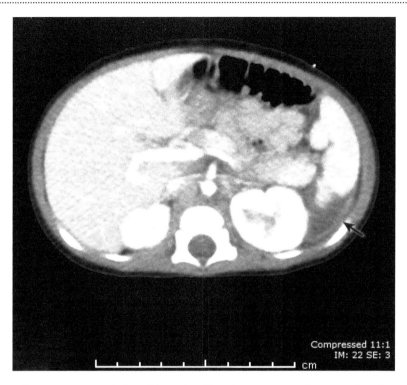

(A) Axial postcontrast CT image demonstrates a complex branching region of low attenuation extending across the spleen, associated with a hypodense fluid collection surrounding the spleen (*arrow*).

■ Differential Diagnosis

- **Splenic laceration:** Diagnosed in the setting of trauma when there is a linear, often branching cleft of hypoattenuation extending into or across the spleen.
- *Splenic cleft:* Congenital clefts of the spleen have a hypodense appearance on postcontrast CT image, but they are generally linear, smooth in contour, and not associated with perisplenic fluid collections.
- *Splenic infarction:* Splenic infarctions appear hypodense, but they are generally wedge shaped and typically are not associated with perisplenic fluid collections.

■ Essential Facts

- Most commonly associated with blunt abdominal trauma.
- High-attenuation fluid around the spleen or in the peritoneal cavity indicative of hemoperitoneum.
- Most patients managed conservatively, but active extravasation or hemodynamic instability may require catheter embolization or splenectomy.

■ Other Imaging Findings

- Can be associated with subcapsular hematoma, which indents the splenic contour.
- Lack of splenic enhancement indicates splenic avulsion.
- Active extravasation appears as a focus in the spleen equal in density to the contrast-opacified blood in the aorta.

✓ Pearls and ✗ Pitfalls

✓ Check for associated injuries, including the liver, pancreas, and ribs.

✗ So-called "tiger stripes" appearance of the spleen in the early arterial phase of contrast enhancement, with alternating bands of hyper- and hypoattenuation corresponding to red and white pulp, should not be mistaken for splenic injury.

Case 75

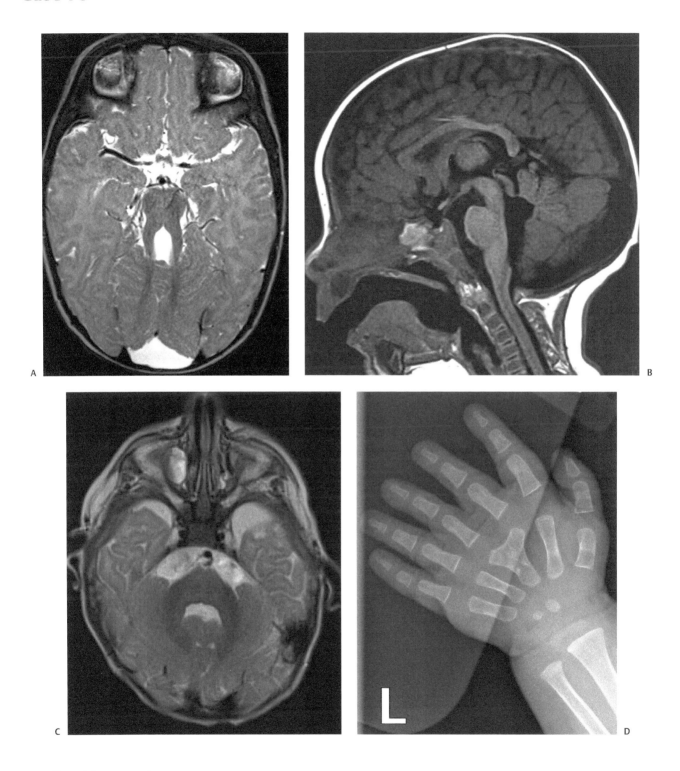

■ Clinical Presentation

A 3-month-old boy with hypotonia and nystagmus.

■ Imaging Findings

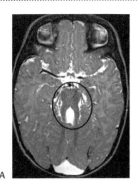 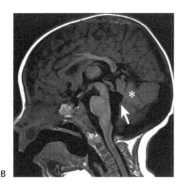 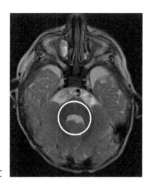 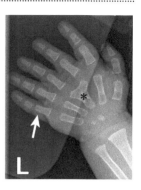

(A) Axial T2-weighted MR image of the brain. The superior cerebellar peduncles are thickened, elongated, parallel, and horizontally oriented. There is a deepened interpeduncular fossa consistent with the molar tooth sign (*circle*). **(B)** Sagittal T1 fluid-attenuated inversion recovery MR image of the brain. There is severe vermian hypoplasia (*asterisk*) with distortion and enlargement of the fourth ventricle (*arrow*). **(C)** Axial T2-weighted MR image of the brain. There is a batwing appearance of the fourth ventricle (*circle*). **(D)** Posteroanterior view of the left hand. On the ulnar aspect of the hand, there is a supernumerary digit with three small phalanges consistent with postaxial polydactyly (*arrow*). In addition, there is a fusion anomaly of the middle metacarpal (*asterisk*).

■ Differential Diagnosis

- **Joubert syndrome:** The molar tooth appearance on the axial images as well as the batwing appearance of the fourth ventricle, vermian hypoplasia, and postaxial polydactyly are all consistent with Joubert syndrome.
- *Cerebellar vermian hypoplasia/atrophy:* In this case, the vermis is small; however, in cerebellar vermian hypoplasia, there would be no other abnormalities. The cerebellar peduncles and midbrain should be normal.
- *Rhombencephalosynapsis:* In rhombencephalosynapsis, the cerebellar hemispheres are fused without a vermis. There would be marked ventriculomegaly and fusion of the thalami.

■ Essential Facts

- Joubert syndrome is a rare autosomal-recessive syndrome characterized by episodic abnormal respiratory patterns, oculomotor findings, hypotonia, ataxia, and developmental retardation.
- The term *Joubert syndrome and related disorders* describes conditions that share the molar tooth sign and some clinical features with Joubert syndrome but also manifest features that may represent a distinct syndrome.

■ Other Imaging Findings

- Diffusion tensor imaging shows absence of fiber decussation in the superior cerebellar peduncles and pyramidal tracts.
- The inferior olivary nucleus is abnormal and there is dysplasia or heterotopia of the cerebellar nuclei.
- Occasionally, ventriculomegaly and dysgenesis of the corpus callosum can be identified.

✓ Pearls and ✗ Pitfalls

- ✓ Associated features include retinal dystrophy, renal cysts, ocular colobomas, occipital encephalocele, hepatic fibrosis, polydactyly, oral hamartomas, and endocrine abnormalities.
- ✗ Molar tooth sign can also be seen in Dekaban–Arima syndrome, cerebellar vermis hypo/aplasia, oligophrenia, congenital ataxia, ocular coloboma, hepatic fibrosis (COACH) syndrome, and Senior–Loken syndrome as well as several others.

Case 76

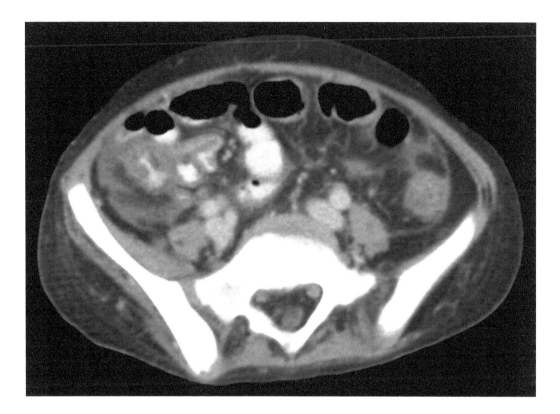

■ Clinical Presentation

A 7-year-old boy being treated for acute myelogenous leukemia who presents with abdominal pain.

■ Imaging Findings

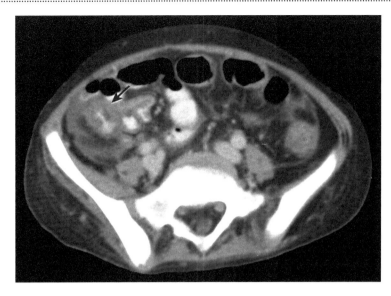

(A) Axial postcontrast CT image demonstrates abnormal wall thickening of the ascending colon (*arrow*) with surrounding fluid and inflammatory changes. Similar changes, although less severe, are seen in the descending colon.

■ Differential Diagnosis

- **Neutropenic colitis:** Typically found in the ascending colon, neutropenic colitis often causes impressive wall thickening and pericolonic inflammatory changes.
- *Ulcerative colitis:* Ulcerative colitis can also cause colonic inflammation and wall thickening, but the inflammation is typically not transmural (except in toxic megacolon), and the history of treatment of leukemia is not typical.
- *Pseudomembranous colitis:* Pseudomembranous colitis, which is associated with *Clostridium difficile* infection, often causes pancolitis, although patients with this disorder generally have a history of treatment with antibiotics but not immunosuppressive therapy.

■ Essential Facts

- Also commonly referred to as typhlitis.
- Likely due to a combination of chemotherapy-related immunosuppression and antibiotic-mediated bacterial overgrowth.
- Can progress to perforation, peritonitis, and sepsis.
- Advanced cases may require surgical resection of affected bowel.

■ Other Imaging Findings

- Radiograph may show a soft tissue mass in the right lower quadrant.
- Radiograph may also demonstrate a partial small-bowel obstruction.
- If high-density fluid is present in the affected bowel wall, it indicates hemorrhage.

✓ Pearls and ✗ Pitfalls

✓ Diagnosis should be considered in any child with neutropenia and right lower quadrant pain.
✗ Contrast enema and endoscopy are contraindicated due to risk of perforation.

Case 77

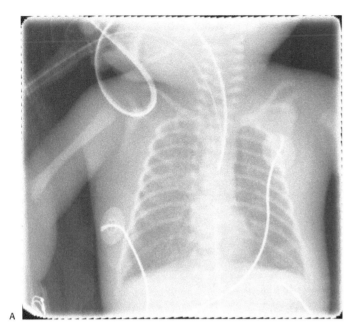
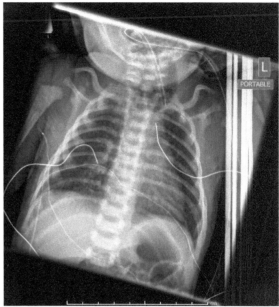

A 1-day-old who chokes with feedings. Multiple attempts to pass an orogastric tube have been unsuccessful.

■ Imaging Findings

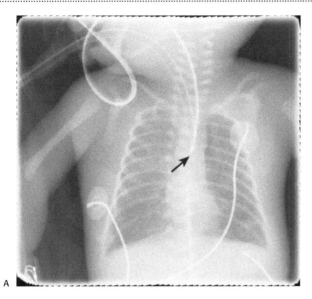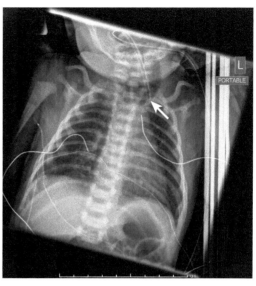

(A) Frontal chest radiograph demonstrates an orogastric tube extending down to the level of the tracheal bifurcation (*arrow*), and there is no gas in the stomach or intestines. An endotracheal tube is at the level of the mid thoracic trachea. **(B)** Different patient, comparison case. Frontal radiograph demonstrates an orogastric tube in a dilated proximal esophageal pouch (*arrow*), but in this case, there is gas in the stomach and intestines.

■ Differential Diagnosis

- ***Esophageal atresia:*** The combination of choking with feedings, inability to pass an orogastric tube, and lack of gas in the stomach and intestines is virtually diagnostic of esophageal atresia without tracheoesophageal fistula.
- *Complication of orogastric tube placement:* Rarely, attempts to pass an orogastric tube may perforate the esophagus, preventing the tube from advancing normally. In such cases, however, gas would still be expected in the stomach and intestines.
- *Vascular ring:* On occasion, a vascular ring may cause sufficient extrinsic mass effect on the esophagus that passage of a tube through the esophagus becomes difficult. However, there should be gas in the stomach and intestines.

■ Essential Facts

- Due to embryologic failure of normal division of foregut into trachea and esophagus.
- When a tracheoesophageal fistula is present, there should be gas in the stomach and intestines; where there is no such fistula, swallowed air cannot reach the stomach.

- Most common types of tracheoesophageal anomalies include type C (esophageal atresia with tracheoesophageal fistula, 85%), type A (esophageal atresia without tracheoesophageal fistula, 10%), and type E (tracheoesophageal fistula without esophageal atresia, 5%).
- Surgical treatment involves primary anastomosis of esophagus and/or ligation of tracheoesophageal fistula.

■ Other Imaging Findings

- Part of the VACTERL association: vertebral, anal, cardiac, tracheoesophageal, renal, and limb anomalies.
- Complications after surgery include anastomotic leak and esophageal dysmotility and stricture.

✓ Pearls and ✗ Pitfalls

- ✓ On chest radiographs, check for signs of congenital heart disease and vertebral anomalies.
- ✓ To detect isolated esophageal atresia, contrast injection directly into the esophagus may be necessary.
- ✗ After surgical repair, signs of anastomotic leak may be subtle.

Case 78

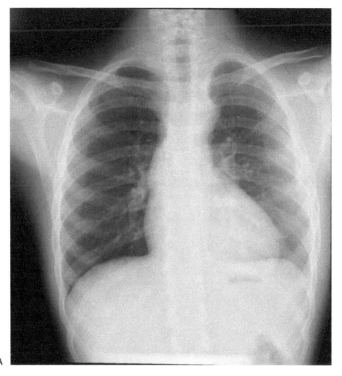

A

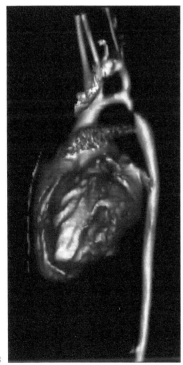

B

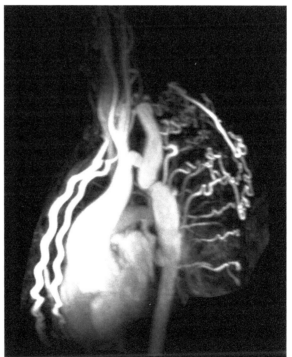

C

▦ Clinical Presentation

A 14-year-old boy with hypertension.

■ Imaging Findings

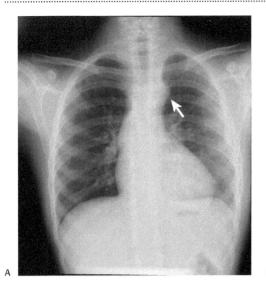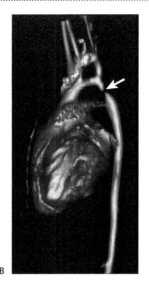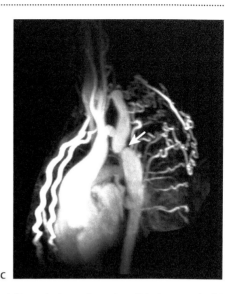

(A) Frontal chest radiograph demonstrates a prominent aortic knob for a patient of this age (*arrow*), a left ventricular configuration of the heart, and mild notching on the undersurface of multiple upper thoracic ribs. **(B)** Three-dimensional CT image of the aorta from a left anterior perspective demonstrates a focal narrowing of the distal aortic arch (*arrow*), just below the junction with the left subclavian artery. **(C)** "Candy-cane" MR image demonstrates the coarctation (*arrow*), dilation of the aortic root, and prominent internal mammary artery and intercostal artery vessels.

■ Differential Diagnosis

- **Coarctation of the aorta:** The findings in this case, including aortic prominence, visualization of the focal narrowing in the arch, rib notching, and prominent collateral vessels, are diagnostic for coarctation.
- *Interrupted aortic arch:* Interrupted aortic arch is associated with complete discontinuity between the aortic arch and descending aorta, with flow to the latter via a patent ductus arteriosus. In this case, the aorta does not appear to be discontinuous. Moreover, the patient is too old to be presenting with an interrupted arch.
- *Pseudocoarctation:* Pseudocoarctation is associated with apparent narrowing at the distal aortic arch, but there is not true obstruction and the prominent collaterals in this case should not be present.

■ Essential Facts

- Some patients are asymptomatic, but those presenting later in childhood and as adults often have hypertension and higher blood pressures in the arms than in the legs.
- Rib notching is generally not seen in the first 5 years of life.
- Can present as an isolated lesion or in association with other anomalies such as bicuspid aortic valve and ventricular septal defect.

■ Other Imaging Findings

- Echocardiography, CT, and MRI can all be used to estimate the degree of stenosis.
- Barium upper gastrointestinal exam may demonstrate "reverse-three" contour of the esophagus, caused by the dilated descending aorta.
- Associated with circle of Willis aneurysms.

✓ Pearls and ✕ Pitfalls

✓ Hypertension is likely due to decreased renal perfusion.
✕ Check for rib notching in patients with unexplained hypertension.

Case 79

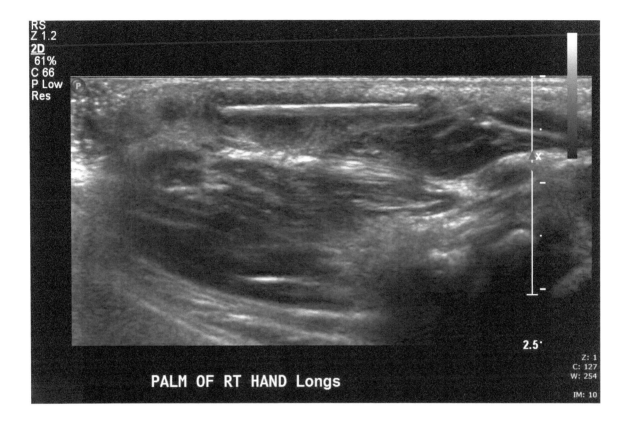

■ Clinical Presentation

A 6-year-old girl with 2 weeks of redness and swelling on the palmar surface of the hand.

■ Imaging Findings

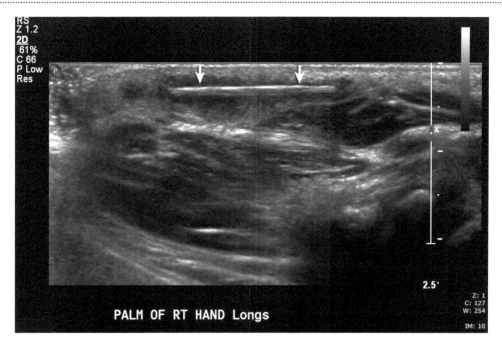

(A) Longitudinal sonographic image of the palmar surface of the right hand reveals a linear hyperechoic object, ~2 cm long, in the soft tissues of the hand (*arrows*). This is essentially diagnostic of a soft tissue foreign body, which turned out to be a splinter of wood.

■ Differential Diagnosis

• **Foreign body:** No other reasonable diagnosis.

■ Essential Facts

• Many foreign bodies are not sufficiently radiopaque to be demonstrated on plain radiographs.
• Such objects are typically easily visualized on ultrasound.
• Ultrasound guidance can also be used for removal.

■ Other Imaging Findings

• Glass and metal are generally visualized on plain radiographs.

• On ultrasound, the shape of a foreign body often appears nonbiologic.
• On MR image, most foreign bodies demonstrate low signal on all sequences, although they are often surrounded by inflammatory changes.

✓ Pearls and ✗ Pitfalls

✓ Ultrasound is generally the imaging modality of choice for superficial foreign bodies.
✗ Normal radiographs do not exclude a foreign body.

Case 80

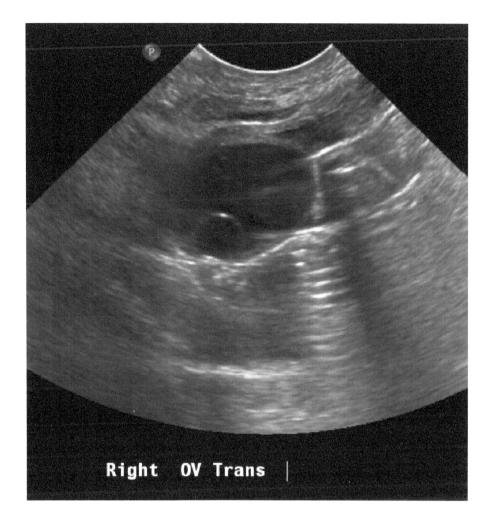

Right OV Trans |

■ Clinical Presentation

A female newborn with an abdominal mass.

■ Imaging Findings

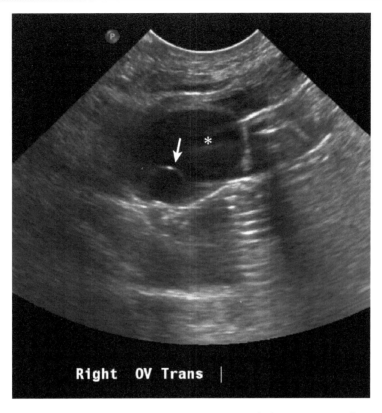

(A) Transverse ultrasound view of the right lower quadrant. There is a cystic structure (*asterisk*) that contains a smaller cyst within it (*arrow*).

■ Differential Diagnosis

- **Simple ovarian cyst:** A cystic structure with a small internal cyst in a newborn female is classic for an ovarian cyst.
- *Meconium pseudocyst:* Although these can present as hypoechoic masses, they typically have an echogenic wall due to calcification.
- *Enteric duplication cyst:* These also can be anechoic cysts, but they usually will have a five-layered wall consisting of alternating hyperechoic and hypoechoic layers referred to as "gut signature."

■ Essential Facts

- A simple ovarian cyst < 2 cm is considered to be a follicle and, therefore, physiologic rather than pathologic. A cyst > 2 cm is considered abnormal.
- Conservative management for simple cysts of < 5 cm is advisable because many will regress spontaneously.

■ Other Imaging Findings

- Simple ovarian cysts are round, thin-walled, anechoic, and unilocular. They can contain a single simple septation.

- A complicated or complex ovarian cyst is heterogeneous and thick-walled and contains multiple septations. It may have fluid–fluid levels or a solid appearance.
- Fetal ovarian cysts can be seen in the third trimester.
- In fetuses with a cystic abdominopelvic mass, fetal MRI can be helpful to delineate organ of origin and the integrity of surrounding organs/tissues.

✓ Pearls and ✗ Pitfalls

✓ The most common abdominal masses in female neonates are ovarian cysts.
✓ A small, round anechoic structure within a larger cyst is called a "daughter cyst" and is pathognomonic for an ovarian cyst.
✓ The incidence of neonatal ovarian cysts rises with increasing placental size, such as in maternal diabetes, preeclampsia, or Rh incompatibility.
✗ In the fetus and newborn, ovarian cysts often appear more often in the abdomen than in the pelvis.

Case 81

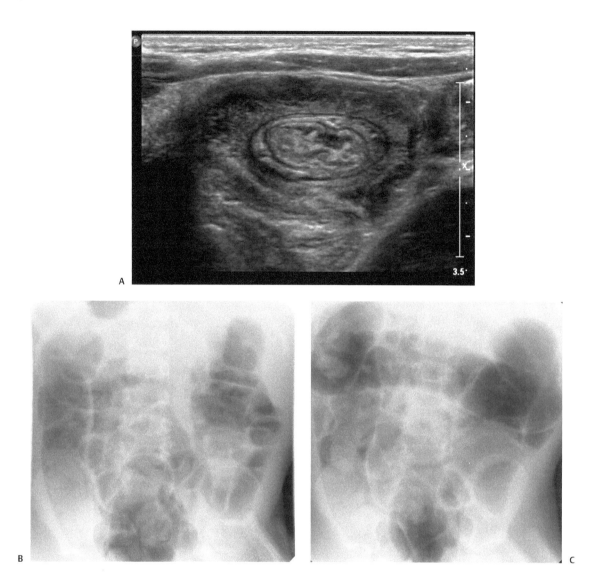

■ Clinical Presentation

A 5-month-old male infant with abdominal pain and bloody stools.

■ Imaging Findings

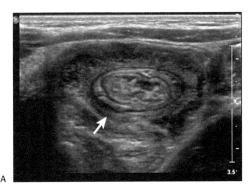

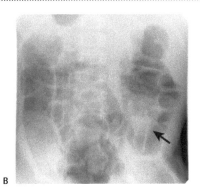

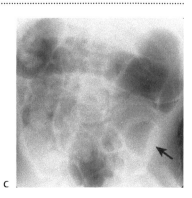

(A) Right lower quadrant ultrasound image demonstrates a classic target sign of intussusception (*arrow*). **(B)** Abdominal fluoroscopic image from an air-contrast enema with the patient in prone position demonstrates air distention of the colon with a soft tissue mass (*arrow*) in the right lower quadrant. **(C)** Another fluoroscopic image from later in the exam (again with the patient in prone position) shows disappearance of the right lower quadrant soft tissue mass (*arrow*) with reflux of air into the small bowel.

■ Differential Diagnosis

- **Intussusception:** The sonographic target sign and the finding of a reducible colonic soft tissue mass are both highly typical of intussusception.
- *Meckel diverticulum:* This lesion can present with abdominal pain and bloody stools, and it can also act as a lead point for intussusception, although most patients with intussusception do not have a Meckel diverticulum and most patients with Meckel diverticula do not develop intussusception. A target sign should not be seen unless intussusception has occurred.
- *Lymphoma:* Patients with small-bowel lymphoma can present with abdominal pain, right lower quadrant mass, and bloody stools, but the target sign should not be present unless intussusception has occurred.

■ Essential Facts

- Most common in the 1st year of life.
- Invagination of proximal bowel into distal bowel, classically ileocolic.
- Inner bowel = intussusceptum; outer bowel = intussuscipiens.
- Liquid contrast or air enema can be both diagnostic and therapeutic.
- Vast majority are idiopathic (no pathologic lead point), most commonly due to lymphoid hyperplasia.
- The longer the intussusception persists, the more likely bowel infarction and perforation become.

■ Other Imaging Findings

- Plain radiographs are not very sensitive but may show right-sided soft tissue mass.
- Ultrasound is highly accurate and should serve as first-line imaging.
- Enema can successfully reduce a majority of intussusceptions.

✓ Pearls and ✗ Pitfalls

- ✓ If a left-side-down decubitus radiograph shows complete filling of the right side of the colon with gas, intussusception is unlikely.
- ✓ Obtaining a good rectal seal is crucial for successful enema reduction.
- ✗ Pneumoperitoneum is a contraindication to reduction attempt.
- ✗ After successful reduction, intussusception recurs in as many as 10% of patients.

Case 82

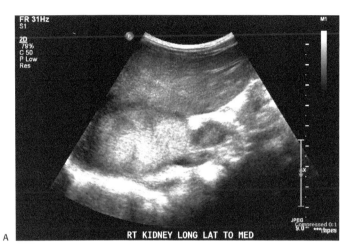

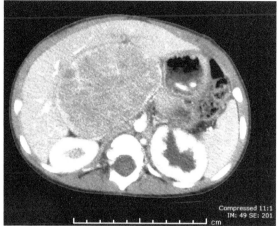

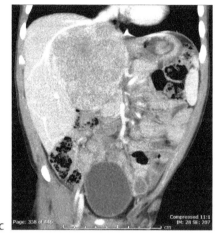

■ Clinical Presentation

A 2-year-old boy with a mass discovered incidentally on renal ultrasound.

■ Imaging Findings

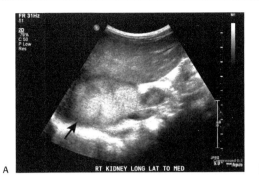 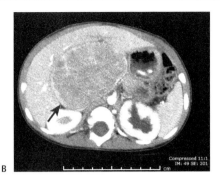 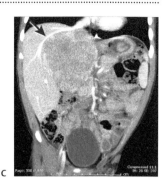

(A) Longitudinal ultrasound image demonstrates a large mass between the liver and the right kidney (*arrow*). **(B)** Axial postcontrast CT image demonstrates a large, well-defined predominantly hypodense mass arising from the liver (*arrow*). **(C)** Coronal postcontrast CT image demonstrates the large, well-defined hypodense mass displacing the right hepatic vein superiorly and to the right (*arrow*).

■ Differential Diagnosis

- **Hepatoblastoma:** Hepatoblastoma is the most common primary hepatic malignancy in the first few years of life, and typically presents as a large, well-defined hypodense mass that displaces or invades hepatic vessels.
- *Hepatocellular carcinoma:* A hepatocellular carcinoma, which represents the most common primary liver malignancy in the 2nd decade of life, could have an identical appearance, but it would be uncommon in a patient this young.
- *Mesenchymal hamartoma:* A relatively common benign hepatic tumor in patients this young, but usually has a multiseptated appearance and includes both solid and cystic components.

■ Essential Facts

- Originates from immature liver precursor cells.
- Associated with markedly elevated α-fetoprotein levels.
- Curable if completely resected, which sometimes requires liver transplantation.

■ Other Imaging Findings

- Relationship to hepatic vessels important in determining resectability.
- Some hepatoblastomas are multifocal.
- Staging includes chest CT to evaluate for pulmonary metastases.

✓ Pearls and ✗ Pitfalls

- ✓ Good response to chemotherapy can make an unresectable tumor resectable.
- ✗ Need to determine whether a right upper quadrant mass in an infant or small child originates from the liver (hepatoblastoma), adrenal gland (neuroblastoma), or kidney (Wilms tumor).

Case 83

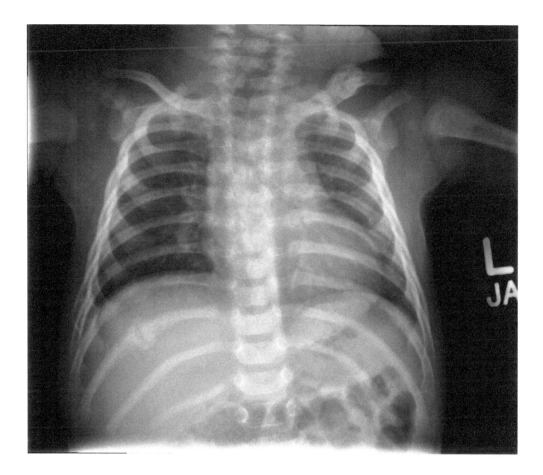

■ Clinical Presentation

An infant with bruising.

■ Imaging Findings

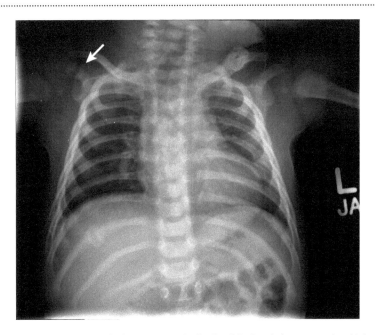

(A) Frontal radiograph demonstrates a healing right scapular fracture (*arrow*), a healing left clavicle fracture, and multiple rib fractures, including a healing fracture of the posterior aspect of the right tenth rib.

■ Differential Diagnosis

- ***Child abuse:*** Scapular fractures have a high specificity for child abuse. Although the clavicular and rib fractures are not so specific, the presence of multiple fractures of different bones is also highly suggestive of child abuse.
- *Osteogenesis imperfecta:* Associated with fragility of the bones, but should be accompanied by other findings such as blue sclerae and wormian bones.
- *Rickets:* Also associated with fragile bones, but it is usually also accompanied by osteopenia and fraying of the metaphyseal margins.

■ Essential Facts

- Fractures thought to be highly specific for abuse include fractures of the scapula, sternum, and vertebral spinous process.
- In difficult cases, CT image of the chest can reliably demonstrate fractures anywhere in the thorax.
- Nuclear medicine bone scans are relatively sensitive for rib fractures.

■ Other Imaging Findings

- Also specific for child abuse are multiple fractures of different ages.
- Additional plain radiographs in different projections often sufficient to identify fractures.
- CT or MR image of the head should be obtained to assess for intracranial injury such as subdural hematoma.

✓ Pearls and ✗ Pitfalls

- ✓ Identification of one suspicious fracture should prompt skeletal survey.
- ✗ Follow-up radiographs can demonstrate initially occult fractures.

Case 84

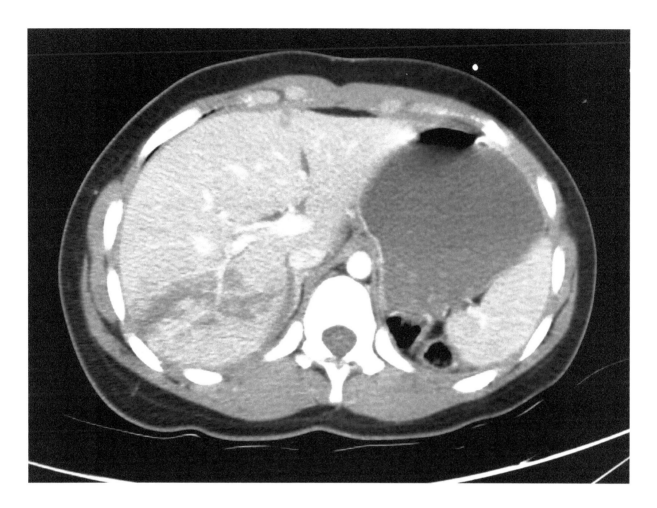

A 15-year-old girl with abdominal pain after a motor vehicle accident.

■ Imaging Findings

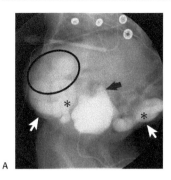 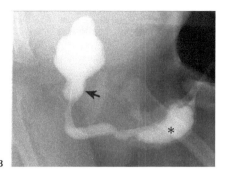 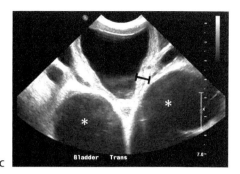

(A) Voiding cystourethrogram (VCUG) view of the abdomen. The flanks are bulging (*white arrows*). The bladder wall is lobular and there is suggestion of a urachal diverticulum (*thick arrow*). There is vesicoureteral reflux into bilateral severely dilated, tortuous ureters (*asterisks*) and a markedly dilated right renal collecting system (*circle*). **(B)** VCUG image of the urethra. The prostatic urethra (*arrow*) is dilated to the membranous urethra. There is a scaphoid megalourethra (*asterisk*). **(C)** Transverse ultrasound view of the bladder. The bladder wall is markedly thickened (*line*) and there is marked dilation of the distal ureters (*asterisks*).

■ Differential Diagnosis

- **Prune belly (Eagle–Barrett or triad) syndrome:** Bulging flanks secondary to dilated, tortuous ureters, absence or hypoplasia of abdominal wall muscles, and a multitude of urinary tract anomalies is consistent with prune belly syndrome.
- *Posterior urethral valves (PUV):* Prune belly syndrome and PUV share the characteristics of a dilated posterior urethra, vesicoureteral reflux, and bladder diverticula. PUV is not associated with bulging flanks, megalourethra, or urachal diverticulum.
- *Anterior urethral valves:* This involves dilation of the urethra proximal to the urethral valves and can cause hydroureteronephrosis. It is not associated with scaphoid configuration of the urethra, absence of abdominal wall musculature, or urachal diverticulum.

■ Essential Facts

- Prune belly syndrome is the triad of hypoplasia of the abdominal muscles, cryptorchidism, and abnormalities of the urinary tract system.
- Eventually, renal insufficiency and renal failure may develop.
- Prune belly syndrome can also be associated with significant pulmonary problems; gastrointestinal anomalies; musculoskeletal anomalies; and, less commonly, cardiovascular anomalies.

■ Other Imaging Findings

- Urinary tract findings may include:
  - Severe bilateral hydroureteronephrosis.
  - Dysplastic and sometimes cystic kidneys.
  - Hypertrophied bladder with diverticula and a urachal diverticulum.
  - Megalourethra, a utricle, or even urethral atresia.
- Bilateral cryptorchidism (intraabdominal testes).

✓ Pearls and ✗ Pitfalls

- ✓ Pseudo–prune belly can occur rarely in girls. Instead of cryptorchidism, girls have genital abnormalities including bicornuate uterus and vaginal atresia.
- ✓ Rarely, prune belly syndrome can be unilateral.
- ✓ Obstructive lesions at the junction of the prostatic and membranous urethra can be seen in ~20%, and this correlates with a poor prognosis.
- ✗ The degree of hydronephrosis does not always correlate with the severity of the abdominal wall deficiency, and the renal parenchyma may be preserved.

Case 86

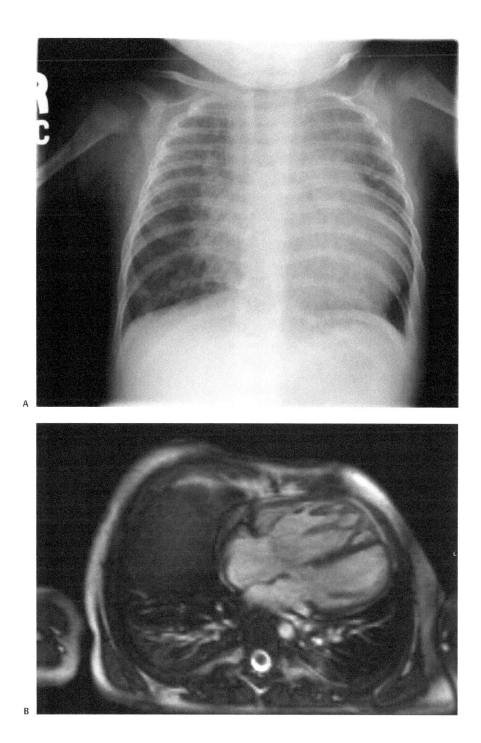

A small 5-year-old girl with respiratory distress.

■ Imaging Findings

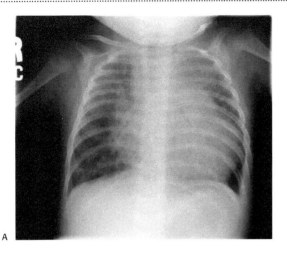
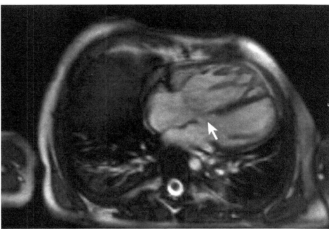

(A) A front chest radiograph demonstrates cardiomegaly and enlargement of the central pulmonary vessels, whose margins appear indistinct, suggesting venous congestion and/or edema. **(B)** Axial MR image demonstrates a defect in the superior portion of the interventricular septum (*arrow*).

■ Differential Diagnosis

- **Ventricular septal defect:** The findings of cardiomegaly, pulmonary vascular enlargement, and vascular congestion/edema are all consistent with this lesion, and the MR image identification of a defect in the interventricular septum establishes the diagnosis.
- *Atrioventricular canal:* Atrioventricular canal is also associated with cardiomegaly and pulmonary vascular enlargement, although patients would usually present earlier in life with more symptoms of left-to-right shunt, and many patients with this lesion have trisomy 21. The MR image is not consistent with atrioventricular canal because only the interventricular septum is involved.
- *Patent ductus arteriosus:* Patent ductus arteriosus also presents with cardiomegaly and enlarged pulmonary vessels, and it could also have this appearance. The defect in the interventricular septum on MR image is not a feature of patent ductus arteriosus.

■ Essential Facts

- Two most common types are membranous (70%), which is located high in the interventricular septum near the aortic valve, and muscular (20%), which is lower in the muscular part of the septum; these defects are often multiple.
- Some muscular defects close spontaneously.

- Noncyanotic because shunt is left to right, involving oxygenated blood.
- Associated with a pansystolic murmur.
- Treatment of larger lesions may include endovascular placement of a closure device or surgical closure.
- Can eventually lead to Eisenmenger syndrome, with the development of pulmonary hypertension and reversal of the shunt to right to left, leading to cyanosis.

■ Other Imaging Findings

- High pulmonary vascular resistance in first days of life tends to reduce the degree of left-to-right shunting, with symptoms and radiographic findings developing later.
- Size of defect is associated with degree of cardiomegaly, pulmonary vascular enlargement, and pulmonary edema.
- MRI enables precise assessment of anatomy and estimation of shunt volume.

✓ Pearls and ✗ Pitfalls

- ✓ Like most forms of congenital heart disease, associated with an increased risk of bacterial endocarditis.
- ✗ With small lesions, chest radiographs may be normal.

Case 87

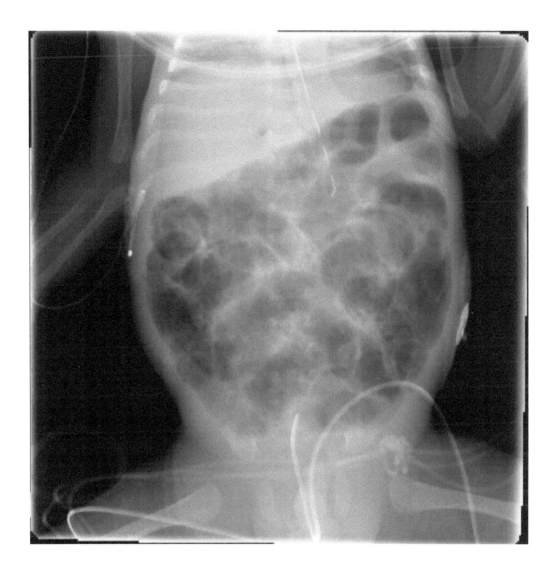

■ Clinical Presentation

A 25-day-old premature boy with feeding intolerance.

■ Imaging Findings

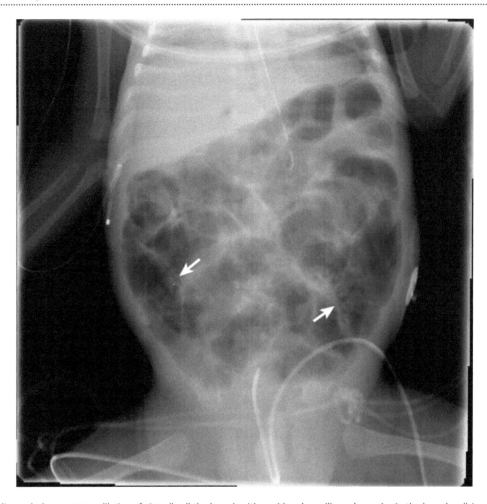

(A) Abdominal radiograph demonstrates dilation of virtually all the bowel, with ovoid and curvilinear lucencies in the bowel wall (*arrows*), representing pneumatosis intestinalis.

■ Differential Diagnosis

- ***Necrotizing enterocolitis:*** In a premature infant with feeding intolerance, pneumatosis intestinalis is strongly suggestive of necrotizing enterocolitis.
- *Sequela of mechanical ventilation:* Bag-mask ventilation and esophageal intubation can both cause abnormal dilation of bowel, although they would not typically be associated with pneumatosis intestinalis.
- *Distal bowel obstruction:* A distal bowel obstruction—for example, from Hirschsprung disease—could cause many segments of abnormally dilated bowel, but it would not typically be associated with pneumatosis intestinalis.

■ Essential Facts

- Strongly associated with prematurity.
- Presentation includes feeding intolerance, abdominal distention, bloody stools, and sepsis.
- Thought to be caused by infection, ischemia, or both.
- Surgery is indicated in patients with pneumoperitoneum.

■ Other Imaging Findings

- Symmetrical distribution of bowel gas.
- Branching lucencies over the liver, indicating gas in the portal venous system.
- Signs of pneumoperitoneum, including central lucency, gas outlining the falciform ligament, gas along the liver on decubitus view, and gas on both sides of bowel wall (Rigler sign).
- Weeks later, patients may develop bowel obstruction from colonic strictures.

✓ Pearls and ✗ Pitfalls

- ✓ In patients too unstable for decubitus radiography, a cross-table lateral radiograph can also detect pneumoperitoneum.
- ✓ Serial abdominal radiographs are typically indicated as surveillance for bowel perforation.
- ✗ Pneumoperitoneum can be difficult to detect on standard supine abdominal radiographs.

Case 88

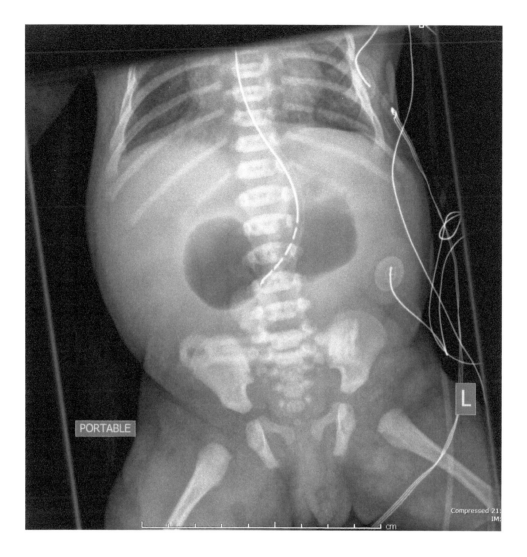

■ Clinical Presentation

A newborn girl with respiratory distress.

■ Imaging Findings

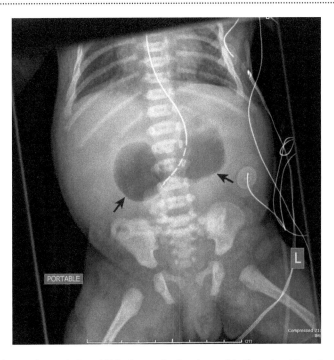

(A) A frontal radiograph of the abdomen demonstrates a bilobed gas collection (*arrows*) in the epigastric region that contains the distal portion of an orogastric tube. No bowel gas is visible distal to this point.

■ Differential Diagnosis

- ***Duodenal atresia:*** This is a classic double bubble, consisting of dilated stomach and duodenum with no distal bowel gas, a classic finding of duodenal atresia, in which the duodenal obstruction is typically complete.
- *Malrotation with midgut volvulus:* Midgut volvulus can present with a high-grade duodenal obstruction. However, because the obstruction is such cases is relatively acute, the proximal duodenum should not be as dilated as in this case, and typically there is at least some distal bowel gas in patients with volvulus.
- *Hypertrophic pyloric stenosis:* Hypertrophic pyloric stenosis can present with a large epigastric gas collection, but it is not a congenital disorder and typically does not present before 2 weeks of life. Also, there is typically only one bubble in hypertrophic pyloric stenosis, whereas this pattern is more consistent with a double bubble.

■ Essential Facts

- Because the duodenum has been obstructed throughout prenatal life, the duodenum is typically quite dilated by the time the patient is born, helping to distinguish duodenal atresia from more acute forms of obstruction such as malrotation with midgut volvulus.
- In contrast to other forms of intestinal atresia (which appear to be related to in utero vascular occlusion), duodenal atresia is thought to be due to a failure of recanalization of the bowel late in embryologic development.

- Approximately 40% of patients with duodenal atresia have trisomy 21, and about one third of patients have malrotation.

■ Other Imaging Findings

- Plain radiography should be sufficient to make the diagnosis (or at least to indicate that the patient needs surgery), and barium studies are not usually indicated.
- On prenatal ultrasound or MR image, the stomach and dilated proximal duodenum are shown to be fluid-filled.
- Because of impaired intestinal resorption of swallowed amniotic fluid, about half of cases are associated with polyhydramnios.

✓ Pearls and ✗ Pitfalls

- ✓ If bowel gas is seen distal to the dilated duodenum, a barium upper gastrointestinal examination may be indicated to assess for other causes such as malrotation and duodenal web.
- ✗ Some patients may develop electrolyte abnormalities that require correction before imaging.

Case 89

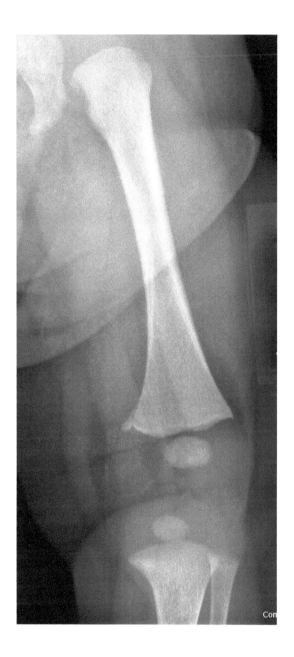

■ Clinical Presentation

A 3-month-old girl with bruising.

■ Imaging Findings

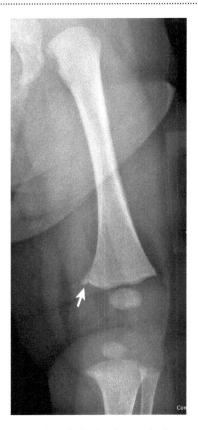

(A) Frontal radiograph of the femur demonstrates a mildly inferolaterally displaced triangular fragment of bone along the distal femoral metaphysis (*arrow*).

■ Differential Diagnosis

- ***Classic metaphyseal lesion:*** Infants cannot generate sufficient force to cause such damage to their bones, and the finding of such a lesion is indicative of child abuse.
- *Metaphyseal spur:* In infants, a prominent triangular shape can involve the distal femoral metaphysis, although there should be no lucent cleft separating it from the bone.
- *Rickets:* Rickets can be associated with a frayed, irregular appearance of the distal metaphysis, but there should be no fracture line separating it from the bone.

■ Essential Facts

- Most common in the distal femur, but also seen in the tibia, humerus, and radius.
- From a different perspective, the same fracture can have a "bucket handle" appearance.
- Thought to be due to shaking or twisting injury.
- Follow-up radiographs in 1 or 2 weeks often show clear periosteal reaction of healing.

■ Other Imaging Findings

- Head CT or MR image may show evidence of intracranial injury, such as subdural hematoma.
- Nuclear medicine bone scan is relatively insensitive due to normal high uptake at physis.
- Follow-up radiographs in 1 to 2 weeks can disclose other injuries that were initially occult.

✓ Pearls and ✗ Pitfalls

✓ Findings suspicious for abuse should be shared with the referring physician.
✗ Failure to obtain follow-up imaging can cause lesions to be missed.

Case 90

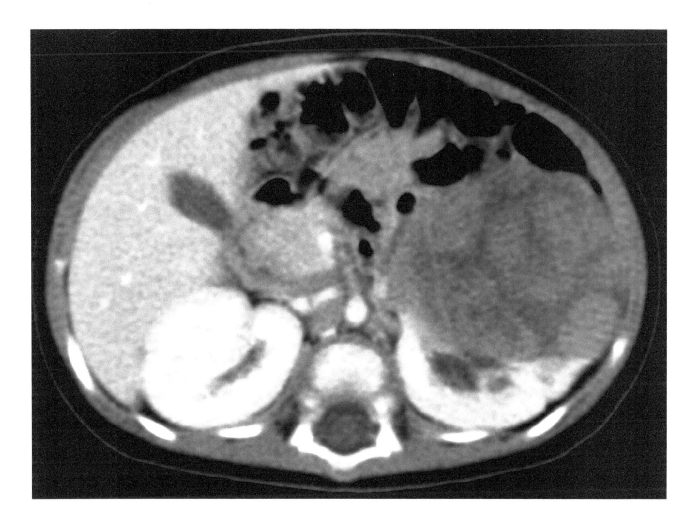

An otherwise healthy 8-month-old boy with hematuria and fever.

■ Imaging Findings

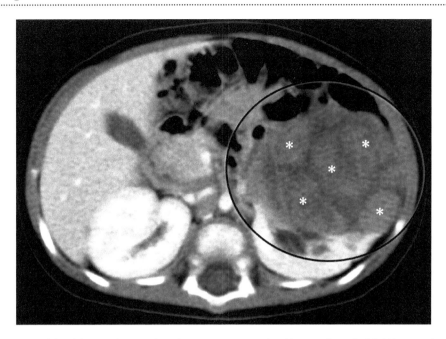

(A) Axial postcontrast CT image of the abdomen. There is a large heterogeneous mass (*circle*) arising from the left kidney. Within the mass, there appear to be round lobules (*asterisks*) separated by hypointense areas.

■ Differential Diagnosis

- **Rhabdoid tumor of the kidney:** A large heterogeneous soft tissue mass involving the renal hilum with tumor lobules separated by low-density areas of necrosis or hemorrhage is consistent with rhabdoid tumor.
- *Wilms tumor:* Wilms tumor can also appear as a large heterogeneous mass and is much more common than rhabdoid tumor. It does not have lobule formation within the tumor.
- *Angiomyolipoma:* Although there is low density in this lesion, it is not low enough to be fat. In children, angiomyolipomas are rare in patients who do not have tuberous sclerosis.

■ Essential Facts

- 80% of rhabdoid tumors occur in children < 2 years of age, with the vast majority being diagnosed between 6 and 12 months of age.
- Associated with synchronous or metachronous primary intracranial tumors (usually midline in the posterior fossa) or early brain metastases.
- Highly aggressive, with most patients presenting with advanced disease.

■ Other Imaging Findings

- Rhabdoid tumors often are composed of lobules separated by dark areas of necrosis or hemorrhage. Linear calcifications often outline the tumor lobules.
- Often have subcapsular fluid collections/hematomas.
- Renal vein and inferior vena cava invasion as well as local invasion is common.
- Most commonly metastasizes to the lungs and less often to the liver, abdomen, brain, lymph nodes, or skeleton.

✓ Pearls and ✗ Pitfalls

✓ Occurs exclusively in children.
✓ May cause hypercalcemia because of elevated parathormone level.
✓ Worst prognosis of all pediatric renal tumors.
✗ Without an associated brain neoplasm, rhabdoid tumor is often indistinguishable from Wilms tumor.
✗ Although subcapsular fluid collections are frequent in rhabdoid tumors, a pediatric renal neoplasm with a subcapsular fluid collection is still more likely to represent Wilms tumor than rhabdoid tumor due to the rarity of rhabdoid tumors.
✗ Most of the pediatric malignant renal tumors, including Wilms, rhabdoid, clear cell sarcoma, and renal cell carcinoma, have similar imaging features. Pathologic evaluation is needed for a definitive diagnosis.

Case 91

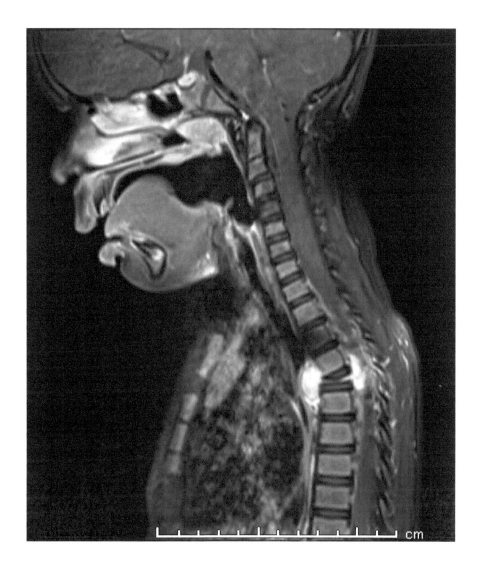

A 5-year-old boy with back pain.

■ Imaging Findings

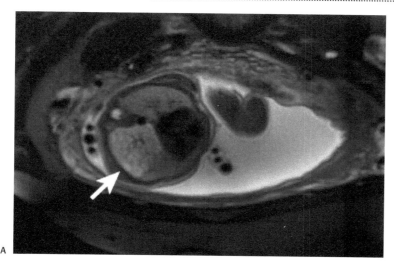
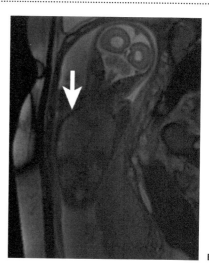

(A) Axial fluid-sensitive MR image demonstrates a large multicystic mass occupying most of the base of the left hemithorax (*arrow*). **(B)** Coronal fluid-sensitive sequence demonstrates that the multicystic mass also extends almost to the top of the left hemithorax (*arrow*).

■ Differential Diagnosis

- ***Congenital pulmonary airway malformation:*** The finding of a multicystic, macrocystic thoracic mass is most characteristic of a congenital pulmonary airway malformation.
- *Congenital diaphragmatic hernia:* Fluid-filled segments of bowel in the thorax can resemble a multicystic thoracic lesion, and the diagnosis would be supported by evidence of peristalsis. However, the left hemidiaphragm appears to be intact and other images clearly demonstrated a normally positioned stomach bubble.
- *Bronchogenic cyst:* Bronchogenic cysts are usually located in closer proximity to the central airways and normally contain a single fluid collection.

■ Essential Facts

- A congenital pulmonary airway malformation is a hamartomatous lesion containing tissue from multiple different pulmonary origins.
- The most common type, accounting for one half to three quarters of lesions, is type I, which arises from a distal bronchus and (postnatally) contains cysts measuring > 3 cm in diameter. The next most common type, type II, represents about one quarter of lesions and consists of smaller cysts measuring between 0.5 and 3 cm in diameter. Type II lesions have the highest association with other anomalies. Type III cysts appear solid.

- Congenital pulmonary airway malformations are often associated with bronchopulmonary sequestration, which consists of nonfunctioning tissue separate from adjacent lung and demonstrates a systemic arterial blood supply.
- These lesions may decrease in size or even disappear over the course of gestation, and they can generally be followed serially by ultrasound.

■ Other Imaging Findings

- Congenital pulmonary airway malformations can be associated with hydrops fetalis, due at least in some cases to mass effect on the heart and congestive heart failure.
- Congenital pulmonary airway malformations can also be associated with polyhydramnios.

✓ Pearls and ✗ Pitfalls

- ✓ Long-term congenital pulmonary airway malformations carry an increased risk of pulmonary malignancies, and even asymptomatic malformations are generally resected in childhood.
- ✓ CT and MRI can be helpful in operative planning, in part to determine whether an apparent congenital pulmonary airway malformation actually represents a hybrid lesion including a component of bronchopulmonary sequestration, as indicated by a systemic arterial supply.

Case Questions and Answers

The questions and answers in the following section are numbered as cases 1 through 100. The questions correspond to the respectively numbered case reviews and are intended to be answered after working through the cases.

▦ Case 1

1. Which of the following conditions is not in the differential diagnosis of an infant with bilious vomiting?
   a) Malrotation with midgut volvulus
   b) Duodenal atresia
   c) Hypertrophic pyloric stenosis
   d) Annual pancreas

The correct answer is (**c**). In contrast to the other choices, in patients with hypertrophic pyloric stenosis, the obstruction is always located proximal to the ampulla of Vater, meaning that bile should not be refluxing back into the stomach to be vomited.

2. In an infant who presents with bilious vomiting, which of the following requires the most urgent surgical treatment?
   a) Malrotation with midgut volvulus
   b) Duodenal atresia
   c) Redundant duodenum
   d) Annular pancreas

The correct answer is (**a**). A redundant duodenum is an anatomic variant that can be mistaken for malrotation but requires no surgical treatment. Of the other choices, the one that requires the most urgent surgical treatment is malrotation with midgut volvulus, because volvulus compromises bowel perfusion and can quickly result in infarction, potentially involving the entire mesenteric small bowel.

▦ Case 2

1. What is one difference between omphalocele and gastroschisis?
   a) In gastroschisis, part of the liver is commonly herniated, whereas in omphalocele, only bowel loops are herniated.
   b) In gastroschisis, the umbilical cord inserts abnormally inferiorly on the abdominal wall, whereas in omphalocele, the umbilical cord inserts normally on the abdominal wall.
   c) In gastroschisis, herniated abdominal contents float freely in the amniotic fluid, whereas in omphalocele, the herniated contents are covered by a membrane.
   d) In gastroschisis, multiple congenital anomalies often can be identified, whereas in omphalocele, associated anomalies are rare.

The correct answer is (**c**). Identification of a membrane covering the herniated abdominal contents is key to distinguishing omphalocele from gastroschisis. In gastroschisis, the cord inserts normally on the abdominal wall, usually to the right of the abdominal wall defect. In omphalocele, the cord inserts on the membrane covering the herniated contents. It is more common for liver to be herniated in omphalocele than in gastroschisis. Gastroschisis is usually an isolated defect, whereas omphalocele is often associated with other structural and chromosomal anomalies.

2. Which of the following is true regarding embryologic development of the gut?
   a) Herniation of bowel loops is considered physiologic until ~20 weeks' gestational age.
   b) Normal rotation of the gut places the superior mesenteric artery on the left and the superior mesenteric vein on the right.
   c) Herniation of liver is considered physiologic until ~13 weeks' gestational age.
   d) Normal rotation of the gut continues until birth.

The correct answer is (**b**). In the normally rotated gut, the superior mesenteric artery is on the left and the vein is on the right. This relationship can often be demonstrated by ultrasound. Of note, a normal relationship does not rule out malrotation. Herniation of loops of bowel is normal until 12 to 13 weeks of gestation; however, no other organs should be seen herniating outside of the abdominal cavity. Normal rotation of the gut is also complete around the time that it reenters the abdomen at 12 weeks of gestation.

▦ Case 3

1. On T2-weighted fetal MR images, which is true regarding the lungs?
   a) Are homogeneously hyperintense relative to the chest wall muscle
   b) Are homogeneously hypointense relative to the chest wall
   c) When compressed, are hyperintense to the chest wall
   d) Become more heterogeneous with advanced gestational age

The correct answer is (**a**). The lungs contain alveolar fluid, causing them to be hyperintense to the chest wall muscle on T2-weighted images. When the lungs become compressed, alveolar fluid is forced out and the signal becomes less intense. The lungs should be homogeneous regardless of gestational age.

2. On fetal MR image, in which of the following lesions should the vessel supplying the lesion typically be seen?
   a) Congenital pulmonary airway malformation
   b) Bronchopulmonary sequestration
   c) Bronchogenic cyst
   d) Congenital diaphragmatic hernia

The correct answer is (**b**). Feeding vessels from the aorta, as seen in sequestrations, can be seen on fetal MR images. The vascular supply of the other lesions is from the pulmonary artery and cannot be delineated on fetal MR images.

■ Case 4

1. Regarding the banana and lemon signs on prenatal ultrasound images of Chiari II malformation, which of the following is correct?
   a) The banana sign refers to the shape of the ventricles.
   b) The banana appearance reverts back to normal after the first trimester.
   c) The lemon sign refers to the shape of the cerebellum.
   d) The lemon sign disappears after 24 weeks' gestational age.

The correct answer is (**d**). The lemon sign refers to the concave or flat shape of the frontal bones of the skull. After 24 weeks, the skull reverts back to its normal ovoid shape. The lemon sign is not exclusive to spina bifida but can be seen in a variety of intracranial abnormalities. The banana sign refers to the wrapping of the cerebellum around the brainstem due to a small posterior fossa. It does not resolve.

2. Which of the following is true regarding gadolinium during pregnancy?
   a) Does not cross the placenta
   b) Is rapidly excreted by the fetal kidneys into the bladder and subsequently into the amniotic fluid
   c) Is routinely used during the third trimester only
   d) Crosses the placenta in such minute quantities that it is not helpful in imaging

The correct answer is (**b**). Gadolinium crosses the placenta and enters into fetal circulation. It is excreted by the fetal kidneys and is seen in the fetal bladder only minutes after maternal administration. Current radiology recommendations discourage the use of gadolinium-based contrast agents during pregnancy because their safety has not been proven.

■ Case 5

1. What is the term used when aspergillosis accumulates in a preexisting cavity?
   a) Angioinvasive aspergillosis
   b) Airway invasive aspergillosis
   c) Saprophytic aspergillosis (aspergilloma)
   d) Allergic bronchopulmonary aspergillosis

The correct answer is (**c**). Aspergilloma refers to a fungus ball that accumulates within a preexisting cavity in the lung. In this case, the aspergillus is not invasive.

2. Which of the following are the two most common underlying causes of saprophytic aspergillosis (aspergilloma)?
   a) Tuberculosis and sarcoidosis
   b) Tuberculosis and emphysema
   c) Emphysema and sarcoidosis
   d) *Staphylococcus aureus* pneumonia and emphysema

The correct answer is (**a**). Tuberculosis and sarcoidosis are the two most common causes of cavities that lead to aspergillomas.

■ Case 6

1. Which of the following is not an iatrogenic etiology of duodenal hematoma?
   a) Anticoagulation
   b) Henoch–Schönlein purpura
   c) Endoscopic biopsy
   d) Cancer chemotherapy

The correct answer is (**b**). Anticoagulation interferes with blood clotting, and cancer chemotherapy can cause thrombocytopenia, both of which increase bleeding risk. Endoscopic biopsy is also associated with duodenal hematoma, especially in patients who are prone to bleeding. Henoch–Schönlein purpura, an immune-complex deposition disorder associated with small-vessel hemorrhage, is also associated with intramural hematomas of the duodenum and other segments of the bowel, but it is not an iatrogenic ("physician-caused") disorder.

2. Which of the following is the most important long-term complication of duodenal hematoma?
   a) Duodenal stricture
   b) Fistula
   c) Chronic pancreatitis
   d) Gallstones

The correct answer is (**a**). Fistula, chronic pancreatitis, and gallstones are not really complications of duodenal hematoma. By contrast, whereas most cases of duodenal hematoma resolve spontaneously over time without long-term sequelae, some develop strictures and associated duodenal obstruction.

■ Case 7

1. Which of the following is true regarding germ cell tumors?
   a) The more solid components a tumor has, the more likely it is to be benign.
   b) The absence of fat on imaging excludes a germ cell tumor from the differential diagnosis.
   c) In order to diagnose a primary malignant mediastinal germ cell neoplasm, it is necessary to exclude a primary gonadal tumor as a source of mediastinal metastases.
   d) Teratoma is the only fat-containing lesion found in the anterior mediastinum.

The correct answer is (**c**). Multiple tumors in the mediastinum can contain fat, including mediastinal lipoma, mediastinal lipomatosis, thymolipoma, and liposarcoma; however, the absence of fat does not exclude a germ cell tumor from the differential diagnosis. The more solid components a germ cell tumor contains, the more likely the tumor is to be malignant.

2. Which of the following would be the least likely to cause an anterior mediastinal mass in a child?
   a) Thymoma
   b) Non-Hodgkin lymphoma
   c) Teratoma
   d) Thymic hyperplasia

The correct answer is (**a**). Thymomas in children are infrequent and only account for 1 to 2% of mediastinal masses in children.

■ Case 8

1. From what portion of the urethra does the utricle arise?
   a) Prostatic
   b) Membranous
   c) Bulbous
   d) Penile

The correct answer is (**a**). A routine voiding cystourethrogram may demonstrate a tiny diverticulum arising from the prostatic urethra called the utricle. It can range from a few millimeters to 1 cm. It is a remnant of the müllerian duct.

2. Which of the following is associated with a patent urachus?
   a) Ureteropelvic junction obstruction
   b) Primary megaureter
   c) Posterior urethral valves
   d) Imperforate anus

The correct answer is (**c**). A persistent patent urachus is associated with congenital lower urinary tract obstructions such as posterior urethral valves or prune belly syndrome. It can also be seen in omphaloceles.

■ Case 9

1. Intramedullary spinal cord astrocytomas are more common in patients with which of the following conditions?
   a) Neurofibromatosis type 1 (NF1)
   b) Neurofibromatosis type 2 (NF2)
   c) von Hippel–Lindau disease (VHL)
   d) Gardner syndrome

The correct answer is (**a**), NF1 is associated with spinal cord astrocytomas, whereas NF2 is associated with spinal cord ependymomas. VHL disease is associated with spinal cord hemangioblastomas. Gardner syndrome is familial colorectal polyposis.

2. Which of the following can occur both intramedullary and in the intradural extramedullary space?
   a) Meningiomas
   b) Astrocytomas
   c) Metastases
   d) Schwannomas

The correct answer is (**c**). Metastases can be found in both compartments. Schwannomas are spinal nerve sheath tumors, and meningiomas arise from the coverings of the spinal cord, so neither would be intramedullary. Astrocytomas arise from glial cells and are intramedullary.

■ Case 10

1. Cysts of which branchial cleft are the most common?
   a) First
   b) Second
   c) Third
   d) Fourth

The correct answer is (**b**). Cysts of the second branchial cleft are the most common. Furthermore, type II is the most common type of second branchial cleft cyst.

The correct answer is (**c**). Pseudospread of the atlas on the axis is also known as a pseudo-Jefferson fracture and may be seen on open-mouth views of the cervical spine. In children up to 4 years of age, up to 6 mm of displacement of the lateral masses relative to the dens is normal. Pseudosubluxation is often seen at C2–C3 and to a lesser extent at C3–C4. Up to 3 mm of anterior wedging of cervical vertebral bodies should not be confused with compression fractures. The absence of lordosis of the cervical spine in children can be normal.

■ Case 18

1. Which of the following is true about normal myelination?
   a) Myelination of the brain is complete at birth.
   b) Normal myelination is not complete until around 18 years of age.
   c) Normal myelination occurs central to peripheral.
   d) The entire corpus callosum is myelinated at birth.

The correct answer is (**c**). Normal myelination progresses from central to peripheral, caudal to rostral, dorsal to ventral, and sensory and then motor. Myelination begins in the 16th week of gestation but does not reach maturity until around 2 years. The corpus callosum may not be completely myelinated until 12 months of age.

2. Which is true about the corpus callosum?
   a) The corpus callosum forms anterior to posterior except for the rostrum, which is formed last.
   b) In partial agenesis of the corpus callosum, the genu is the missing portion.
   c) In complete callosal agenesis, the lateral ventricles are fused.
   d) In complete callosal agenesis, the cingulate sulcus and gyrus are always normal.

The correct answer is (**a**). Callosal agenesis may be partial or complete. When partial, the splenium and rostrum are the missing portions. In complete agenesis, the corpus callosum, cingulate sulcus, and cingulate gyrus are absent. In addition, in complete agenesis, the lateral ventricles are widely spaced and parallel. The occipital horns are dilated (colpocephaly) and the frontal horns are often small and pointed.

■ Case 19

1. Because of their location and signal intensity, Deflux injections can be mistaken for which of the following on MR images?
   a) Seminal vesical cysts
   b) Stones at the ureterovesical junction (UVJ)
   c) Thrombus
   d) Solid bladder mass

The correct answer is (**a**). After Deflux is injected at the UVJ, it may migrate along Waldeyer's sheath to a more extravesical location, mimicking seminal vesical cysts. Without a thorough patient history, they can be difficult to distinguish from one another. On CT images, calcified Deflux injections may mimic stones. Because Deflux has a T2 bright appearance, it would not be confused with a solid bladder mass or thrombus.

2. Without a careful patient history, Deflux injections can be mistaken for which of the following on voiding cystourethrograms (VCUGs)?
   a) Debris within the bladder
   b) Stones at the UVJ
   c) Ureteroceles
   d) Seminal vesical cysts

The correct answer is (**c**). In retrospective studies, VCUGs demonstrated Deflux as filling defects similar to ureteroceles on early filling images in ~30% of patients. Knowing the patient's history as well as the presence or absence of duplicated collecting systems can help to differentiate.

■ Case 20

1. When ependymomas arise supratentorially, where is the most common location?
   a) Along the optic nerve
   b) Within the lateral ventricle
   c) In the periventricular white matter
   d) In the thalamic nuclei

The correct answer is (**c**). Unlike posterior fossa ependymomas, most supratentorial ependymomas are extraventricular. They are often located near the ventricular margins and can extend into the ventricular system.

2. In which posterior fossa tumor is cerebrospinal fluid (CSF) seeding to the spinal cord and meninges most common?
   a) Medulloblastoma
   b) Pilocytic astrocytoma
   c) Brainstem glioma
   d) Ependymoma

The correct answer is (**a**). In ~30% of cases of medulloblastoma, there is CSF seeding to the spinal cord and meninges. Contrast-enhanced imaging of the entire neuraxis should be obtained.

Case 21

1. Which of the following is not a complication of duodenal perforation?
   a) Peritonitis
   b) Sepsis
   c) Pancreatitis
   d) Abscess

The correct answer is (**c**). Peritonitis, abscess, and sepsis are all well-known complications of intestinal perforation. Although pancreatitis can follow trauma in which both the duodenum and pancreas are injured, pancreatitis is not a complication of duodenal perforation itself.

2. Which portion of the duodenum is not retroperitoneal?
   a) First
   b) Second
   c) Third
   d) Fourth

The correct answer is (**a**). The second, third, and fourth portions of the duodenum are retroperitoneal, but the first portion, also called the duodenal bulb, is intraperitoneal.

Case 22

1. Which of the following is true about extralobar sequestration?
   a) Approximately 20% arise within or below the hemidiaphragm.
   b) It is an acquired lesion.
   c) It is not associated with other congenital anomalies.
   d) The most common location is the right lower lobe.

The correct answer is (**a**). The most common location of an extralobar sequestration is the left lower lobe, although 20% lay below or within the hemidiaphragm. It is thought to be a congenital lesion (whereas intralobar is sometimes argued to be acquired); 65% of extralobar sequestrations are associated with other anomalies such as congenital pulmonary airway malformations, congenital heart disease, congenital diaphragmatic hernia, and scimitar syndrome.

2. Intralobar sequestration is different from extralobar sequestration in which of the following ways?
   a) Intralobar sequestration has its own pleural covering, whereas extralobar does not.
   b) The feeding vessel to the intralobar sequestration comes from the thoracic aorta, whereas the feeding vessel to the extralobar sequestration can come from the abdominal aorta.
   c) Intralobar sequestrations usually drain via the pulmonary veins, whereas extralobar drain via systemic veins.
   d) Intralobar sequestrations communicate with the tracheobronchial tree, but extralobar do not.

The correct answer is (**c**). Intralobar sequestrations usually drain via the pulmonary veins, whereas extralobar drain via systemic veins. Extralobar sequestrations have their own pleural covering, but intralobar do not. The feeding vessel to either type of sequestration can arise from any part of the aorta. Neither type of sequestration communicates with the tracheobronchial tree.

Case 23

1. On a normal breast ultrasound image, which of the following is the correct order from hypoechoic to hyperechoic?
   a) Fibrous tissue, fat, glandular tissue
   b) Glandular tissue, fat, fibrous tissue
   c) Fibrous tissue, glandular tissue, fat
   d) Fat, glandular tissue, fibrous tissue

The correct answer is (**d**). On an ultrasound image, the fat in normal breast parenchyma is hypoechoic, glandular tissue is intermediate, and fibrous tissue is echogenic.

2. A juvenile or cellular fibroadenoma is a subtype of fibroadenoma that has which characteristic?
   a) Undergoes markedly rapid growth
   b) Involutes spontaneously
   c) Has a high malignancy potential
   d) Contains multiple small calcifications

The correct answer is (**a**). A juvenile or cellular fibroadenoma is a subtype of fibroadenoma that frequently undergoes rapid growth. They most often occur in African American adolescent girls. They can be multiple or bilateral. Skin ulceration or distended superficial veins may be noted. Juvenile fibroadenomas can be uniformly hypoechoic or may have internal slender, fluid-filled clefts.

Case 24

1. Which of the following is the most common tumor of the pineal region?
   a) Pineoblastoma
   b) Pineocytoma
   c) Germinoma
   d) Teratoma

The correct answer is (**c**). Germ cell tumors are the most common pineal region tumor. Of the germ cell tumors, germinoma is more common than teratoma and makes up 50 to 70% of all pineal neoplasms.

2. The differential diagnosis for a thick and enhancing pituitary infundibulum includes germinoma and what other entity?
   a) Sturge–Weber syndrome
   b) Mucopolysaccharidoses
   c) Osteomyelitis
   d) Langerhans cell histiocytosis

The correct answer is (**d**). The differential diagnosis for a thickened, enhancing infundibulum includes germinoma, Langerhans cell histiocytosis, lymphocytic hypophysitis, sarcoidosis, meningitis, lymphoma, metastases, glioma, and primitive neuroectodermal tumor.

Case 25

1. The difference between semilobar holoprosencephaly and lobar holoprosencephaly is that in *lobar* holoprosencephaly, which of the following occurs?
   a) The corpus callosum is hypoplastic in lobar holoprosencephaly.
   b) The thalami are not fused in lobar holoprosencephaly.
   c) The falx is absent in lobar holoprosencephaly.
   d) There is interdigitation of the falx in lobar holoprosencephaly.

The correct answer is (**b**). The corpus callosum can be hypoplastic in both lobar and semilobar holoprosencephaly. The thalami are not fused in lobar holoprosencephaly but are partially or completely fused in semilobar holoprosencephaly. The falx is present in lobar holoprosencephaly but is rudimentary in semilobar holoprosencephaly. Interdigitation of the interhemispheric fissure is not an issue in holoprosencephaly.

2. Semilobar holoprosencephaly may be accompanied by which facial defect?
   a) Proboscis
   b) Cyclopia
   c) Cleft lip
   d) Mono nostril

The correct answer is (**c**). Cleft lip and hypotelorism are both associated with semilobar holoprosencephaly. More severe facial anomalies such as the others listed are associated with alobar holoprosencephaly.

Case 26

1. Which of the following congenital cardiac anomalies is associated with an "egg-on-a-string" appearance of the heart?
   a) Tetralogy of Fallot
   b) Coarctation of the aorta
   c) Transposition of the great arteries
   d) Ventricular septal defect

The correct answer is (**c**). The position of the transposed great arteries in the same sagittal plane leads to a particularly narrow mediastinal waist, which, combined with cardiomegaly, produces the "egg-on-a-string" appearance of transposition of the great arteries.

2. What key feature distinguishes L-transposition of the great arteries from D-transposition of the great arteries?
   a) Dextrocardia
   b) Atrioventricular discordance
   c) Levocardia
   d) Levoposition of the heart

The correct answer is (**b**). As in D-transposition, the great vessels are connected to the wrong ventricles, but in addition, the atria are connected to the wrong ventricles.

Case 27

1. On imaging, what is the difference between Wilms tumor and mesoblastic nephroma?
   a) Wilms tumor tends to be infiltrative and surrounds adjacent structures.
   b) Wilms tumor typically is heavily calcified.
   c) Mesoblastic nephroma rarely invades the renal vein.
   d) Mesoblastic nephroma is usually metastatic at the time of diagnosis.

The correct answer is (**c**). Although the cellular variant of mesoblastic nephroma can invade the perinephric fat and connective tissue it tends to spare the renal pelvis and vascular pedicle. Invasion of the renal vein is common in Wilms tumor. Neither Wilms tumor nor mesoblastic nephroma infiltrate is heavily calcified. Mesoblastic nephroma rarely metastasizes, although it can metastasize to the lung, brain, or bones. It is not uncommon for Wilms tumor to metastasize to the lungs.

2. Which of the following is true of mesoblastic nephroma?
   a) It is the most common pediatric renal tumor.
   b) It has the best prognosis if resected before 2 years of age.
   c) Peak age of occurrence is 3 years.
   d) Imaging can range from completely solid to predominately cystic masses, and the tumor can locally invade perinephric tissues.

The correct answer is (**b**). Mesoblastic nephroma is the most common solid renal tumor in the neonate. Wilms tumor is the most common pediatric renal mass, and the peak age of incidence of Wilms tumor is 3 to 4 years. The diagnosis of mesoblastic nephroma is usually made in the antenatal period or immediately after birth. It has the best prognosis if resected in the first 6 months of life; however, the prognosis is good overall.

■ Case 28

1. A patient has a testicular mass and an elevated α-fetoprotein (AFP). Which is the most likely diagnosis?
   a) Teratoma
   b) Yolk sac tumor
   c) Hematoma
   d) Lymphoma

The correct answer is (**b**). AFP is elevated in 90% of patients with yolk sac tumors. The one exception is in infants because AFP levels in healthy infants are quite high. Thus, during the first 6 months of life, AFP levels overlap among patients with yolk sac tumors and benign tumors. Lactate dehydrogenase can also be elevated in patients with yolk sac tumor, although this is the least specific.

2. When a testicular tumor metastasizes to lymph nodes, where are the first lymph nodes affected located?
   a) Ipsilateral groin
   b) Contralateral groin
   c) Intrascrotal, extratesticular
   d) Para-aortic/retroperitoneal

The correct answer is (**d**). Right-sided testicular tumors involve pericaval nodes. Left-sided tumors typically metastasize to the preaortic and left para-aortic nodes.

■ Case 29

1. Which is the most common central nervous system tumor in neurofibromatosis type 1 (NF1)?
   a) Optic pathway glioma
   b) Juvenile pilocytic astrocytoma
   c) Brainstem glioma
   d) Spinal astrocytoma

The correct answer is (**a**). Although all of those tumors can occur in NF1, optic gliomas are the most common.

2. What is a characteristic finding in the skull in NF1?
   a) Frontal bossing
   b) Micrognathia
   c) Sphenoid wing dysplasia
   d) Zygomatic arch hypoplasia

The correct answer is (**c**). Sphenoid bone dysplasia is uncommon, but it manifests as hypoplasia of the greater and lesser sphenoid wings with enlargement of the middle cranial fossa. It can be an isolated finding or occur in conjunction with a plexiform neurofibroma. It is characteristic of, but not pathognomonic for, NF1.

■ Case 30

1. Which radioisotope has avid uptake by neural crest tumors?
   a) Sestamibi
   b) Thallium chloride
   c) Meta-iodobenzylguanidine (MIBG)
   d) Disofenin iminodiacetic acid (DISIDA)

The correct answer is (**c**). MIBG is a neurotransmitter precursor in any neuroectodermal tumor and can be used to image neuroblastoma, carcinoid, pheochromocytoma, and paraganglioma. Sestamibi and thallium chloride are used in cardiac imaging, and DISIBA is used in hepatobiliary imaging.

2. Which of the following metastases can occur in neuroblastoma stage IV-S disease?
   a) Bone marrow
   b) Bone cortex
   c) Bony orbit
   d) Local vertebral body invasion

The correct answer is (**a**). Patients with neuroblastoma can be considered stage IV-S if they are younger than 1 year of age at diagnosis as long as their metastatic disease is confined to bone marrow, liver, and skin. Stage IV-S may spontaneously regress.

■ Case 31

1. Which of the following disorders is not associated with an increased risk of malrotation?
   a) Heterotaxy syndromes
   b) Omphalocele
   c) Meconium plug syndrome
   d) Congenital diaphragmatic hernia

The correct answer is (**c**). In heterotaxy syndromes, omphalocele, and congenital diaphragmatic hernia, the small bowel is typically abnormally located during in utero life, leading to abnormal fixation. By contrast, meconium plug syndrome is not associated with abnormal bowel location.

2. Even in a patient without malrotation, the duodenal junction may be displaced caudally and to the right due to which condition?
   a) Splenic mass
   b) Distended stomach
   c) Dilated small bowel
   d) All of the above

The correct answer is (**d**). All of the choices offered may displace the duodenal–jejunal junction inferiorly and to the right, even in a patient without malrotation. Of course, the same also applies in reverse—an abnormally located duodenal–jejunal junction may be displaced into apparently normal position by a mass or intestinal distention.

■ Case 32

1. Which is true in reference to mammography in children?
   a) It is the exam of choice to exclude breast cancer.
   b) It is contraindicated because of the increased risk of radiation-induced malignant changes in the young, glandular breast.
   c) It is favored over ultrasound because ultrasound does not penetrate fibroglandular breast tissue.
   d) It is favored in children with Tanner stage I and II because of its ease of identifying normal breast tissue.

The correct answer is (**b**). In contrast to adults, mammography is contraindicated in all children because of the extremely low risk of breast cancer in the pediatric population and because of poor image quality due to the dense fibroglandular tissue. There is an increased risk of radiation-induced malignant changes.

2. Which is true in reference to malignant breast lesions in children?
   a) They are most commonly adenocarcinoma.
   b) They are more common than benign breast lesions.
   c) They have variable and nonspecific ultrasound characteristics that are similar to characteristics seen in adults.
   d) They are more likely to be primary rather than secondary lesions.

The correct answer is (**c**). Malignant breast lesions in children are very rare. They are more likely to be secondary to metastatic or disseminated tumors such as lymphoma, leukemia, rhabdomyosarcoma, and neuroblastoma. Phyllodes tumor is the most common malignant breast mass in children.

■ Case 33

1. One third of pilocytic astrocytomas in the optic chiasm are associated with which syndrome?
   a) PHACES (posterior fossa malformations, hemangiomas, arterial anomalies, cardiac defects, eye abnormalities, sternal cleft, and supraumbilical raphe)
   b) Turcot
   c) Neurofibromatosis type 1 (NF1)
   d) Neurofibromatosis type 2

The correct answer is (**c**). Cerebellar pilocytic astrocytoma is associated with PHACES and Turcot syndrome as well as Ollier syndrome; however, pilocytic astrocytomas in the optic chiasm are associated most frequently with NF1.

2. Of the following four infratentorial tumors, which is most likely to be found in the cerebellar hemispheres?
   a) Medulloblastoma
   b) Juvenile pilocytic astrocytoma (JPA)
   c) Brainstem glioma
   d) Ependymoma

The correct answer is (**b**). JPA arises in the cerebellar hemisphere and displaces the fourth ventricle rather than occurring within it. Medulloblastoma fills the fourth ventricle and enlarges it. An ependymoma is a "plastic" tumor that arises in the fourth ventricle but often extends out the fourth ventricle foramina. A brainstem glioma arises in the brainstem.

■ Case 34

1. Which lesion is least likely to be confused with pleuropulmonary blastoma?
   a) Cystic pulmonary adenomatoid malformation (CPAM)
   b) Ewing sarcoma
   c) Wilms tumor metastases
   d) Primitive neuroectodermal tumor

The correct answer is (**c**). Because pleuropulmonary blastoma is a rare tumor, there are multiple tumors on the differential diagnosis. The purely cystic type of pleuropulmonary blastoma (type I) is impossible to distinguish from type I CPAM. The solid forms of pleuropulmonary blastoma (types II and III) are often difficult to distinguish from other solid tumors in the chest. Wilms tumor metastases are usually smaller and multiple.

2. Which is the most common solid lung neoplasm in a child?
   a) Metastatic disease
   b) Pleuropulmonary blastoma
   c) Bronchogenic carcinoma
   d) Carcinoid tumor

The correct answer is (**a**). A solid lesion in the lungs is 12 times more likely to be a metastatic lesion than a primary lung neoplasm. The two most common primary tumors in children are pleuropulmonary blastoma and carcinoid tumor. The two most common metastases to the lung are Wilms tumor and osteosarcoma. The common types of lung cancer in adults are rare in children.

■ Case 35

1. Which of the following is most likely to be found in a patient with Poland syndrome?
   a) Bilateral absence of breast tissue
   b) Syndactyly
   c) Preauricular tags
   d) Ipsilateral focal femoral defect

The correct answer is (**b**). Poland syndrome is unilateral and associated with ipsilateral upper extremity anomalies.

2. Which of the following is least likely to cause a unilateral hyperlucent hemithorax?
   a) Pneumothorax
   b) Thoracic scoliosis
   c) Air-trapping
   d) Aspiration

The correct answer is (**d**). The differential for a unilateral hyperlucent lung includes patient positioning, scoliosis, chest wall defects, pneumothorax and contralateral pleural effusion, air-trapping, and differences in perfusion between lungs.

■ Case 36

1. Which of the following is not a cause of tarsal coalition?
   a) Tumor
   b) Trauma
   c) Congenital
   d) Arthritis

The correct answer is (**a**). Although most coalitions are congenital, trauma, arthritis, and infection can all result in coalition. Tumors, by contrast, are not a cause of coalition.

2. Which of the following types of coalition tends to present latest in childhood?
   a) Calcaneonavicular
   b) Talocalcaneal
   c) Talonavicular
   d) Answers b and c

The correct answer is (**b**). Talonavicular coalitions usually present in the first decade of life, calcaneonavicular coalitions usually present around 10 years of age, and talocalcaneal coalitions usually present in the mid-teen years.

■ Case 37

1. In acute pyelonephritis, power Doppler imaging may show which of the following?
   a) Focal areas of increased perfusion
   b) Wedge-shaped areas with decreased perfusion
   c) Diffusely increased perfusion of the renal cortex
   d) Diffusely decreased perfusion of the renal cortex

The correct answer is (**b**). Power Doppler imaging in acute infection may show wedge-shaped areas with decreased perfusion. Color Doppler is less sensitive than power Doppler for this finding.

2. What is the disadvantage of using renal cortical scintigraphy for detecting pyelonephritis?
   a) Tc-99m dimercaptosuccinic acid (DMSA) also is excreted in the bladder, making infection in the bladder difficult to detect.
   b) Tc-99m DMSA uptake is only minimally increased in active infection, making focal infection difficult to differentiate from normal kidney.
   c) Tc-99m DMSA cannot distinguish active disease from scarred areas because both produce photopenic areas.
   d) Tc-99m DMSA cannot distinguish active disease from the renal collecting system because both produce photopenic areas.

The correct answer is (**c**). Renal cortical scintigraphy can be done with technetium labeled with DMSA or glucoheptonate (GHA). These agents cannot discriminate between active disease, abscess, and scarring because all will cause photopenic defects. Furthermore, even in the absence of scarring, photopenic defects may not regain a normal appearance for up to 5 months.

The correct answer is (**d**). The most common site of rhabdomyosarcoma in children is the head and neck. The genitourinary tract is the second most common site of rhabdomyosarcoma in children.

2. What is the only type of genitourinary rhabdomyosarcoma that tends to occur in adolescents?
    a) Prostatic
    b) Bladder
    c) Paratesticular
    d) Cervical

The correct answer is (**c**). Paratesticular tumors are the only type of genitourinary rhabdomyosarcomas that tend to occur in older children/adolescents. The peak age of rhabdomyosarcoma is 3 to 6 years.

■ Case 51

1. The normal conus medullaris is virtually always positioned above which disk space?
    a) T12–L1
    b) L1–2
    c) L2–3
    d) L3–4

The correct answer is (**c**). The normal conus medullaris is virtually always positioned above L2–L3. The cord usually ends between T12 and L2, and if it is found to terminate below the L2–3 disk space, it is considered abnormal. In the setting of tethered cord with the absence of a spinal dysraphism, abnormities of the filum terminale, including fibrolipoma and tight filum terminale syndrome, are common causes.

2. A small cyst in which area of the spinal cord can be a normal variant?
    a) Cervical spinal cord
    b) Thoracic spinal cord
    c) Lumbar spinal cord
    d) Filum terminale

The correct answer is (**d**). A filar cyst, also called a ventriculus terminalis, may be found at the transition of the tip of the conus medullaris to the origin of the filum terminale. It may be as long as 10 mm and as wide as 4 mm. It is an incidental finding and has no clinical significance.

■ Case 52

1. On a sonogram for suspected hypertrophic pyloric stenosis, which of the following is the best landmark for locating the pyloric channel?
    a) The gastroesophageal junction
    b) The gallbladder
    c) The superior mesenteric artery
    d) The head of the pancreas

The correct answer is (**b**). The gastroesophageal junction, superior mesenteric artery, and head of the pancreas are not useful anatomic landmarks for locating the pyloric channel. By contrast, the pylorus is typically located close to the gallbladder.

2. In general, the threshold for diagnosing hypertrophic pyloric stenosis is a pylorus that measures which of the following dimensions?
    a) Muscle thickness of 1 mm and channel length of 12 mm
    b) Muscle thickness of 2 mm and channel length of 14 mm
    c) Muscle thickness of 3 mm and channel length of 16 mm
    d) Muscle thickness of 4 mm and channel length of 18 mm

The correct answer is (**c**). Using lower thresholds for muscle thickness and channel length increases sensitivity but decreases specificity, whereas higher thresholds decrease sensitivity but increase specificity.

■ Case 53

1. Which of the following is not a feature of scimitar syndrome?
    a) Anomalous pulmonary venous drainage
    b) Lower lobe mass
    c) Hypoplasia of the right lung
    d) Systemic arterial supply to a portion of the right lung

The correct answer is (**b**). Anomalous pulmonary draining, pulmonary hypoplasia, and systemic arterial supply to a portion of the lung are all features of scimitar syndrome. By contrast, a lower lobe mass would be characteristic of another condition that can be associated with anomalous pulmonary venous drainage—pulmonary sequestration.

2. Which age of presentation of scimitar syndrome is associated with the worst prognosis?
    a) Infancy
    b) Older childhood
    c) Adolescence
    d) Adulthood

The correct answer is (**a**). Because the degree of left-to-right shunting and associated anomalies is generally most severe in patients who present early with scimitar syndrome, presentation in infancy is associated with the worst prognosis.

Case 54

1. Which of the following is not a common imaging feature of ulcerative colitis?
    a) Thumbprinting
    b) Fistula
    c) "Lead-pipe" colon
    d) "Collar-button" ulcers

The correct answer is (**b**). Thumbprinting, "lead-pipe" colon, and "collar-button" ulcers (due to lateral spread of ulcers in the submucosa) are all common imaging features of ulcerative colitis. Fistula formation, on the other hand, is typical of Crohn disease, which is a transmural inflammatory process, as opposed to ulcerative colitis, which does not extend all the way through the bowel wall, making fistula formation unlikely.

2. Which of the following is not an important goal of radiologic imaging in pediatric patients with suspected inflammatory bowel disease?
    a) Determine disease distribution
    b) Assess for complications
    c) Differentiate Crohn disease from ulcerative colitis
    d) Assess treatment response
    e) All of the above are correct

The correct answer is (**e**). In patients with suspected inflammatory bowel disease, radiologic imaging is used to determine disease extent and distribution, differentiate Crohn disease from ulcerative colitis, and assess for complications and treatment response.

Case 55

1. Which of the following is true regarding the thymus?
    a) The normal thymus can extend into the neck and posterior to the superior vena cava.
    b) On fluoroscopy, the thymus should remain fixed in position.
    c) Scattered calcifications are common in the normal thymus.
    d) A normal thymus can compress vessels.

The correct answer is (**a**). A retrocaval thymus is a normal variant in which the thymus extends posteriorly between the superior vena cava and great arteries. On fluoroscopy, the thymus changes contour and size with respiration. The normal thymus should not contain calcifications or compress vessels or the airway.

2. Which of the following is true regarding lymphoma in children?
    a) Lymphoma is the most common middle mediastinal mass in children.
    b) Fluorodeoxyglucose (FDG)-positron emission tomography (PET) CT images can help delineate scar tissue/fibrosis from residual disease after treatment.
    c) Lymphoma that is early PET responsive has a poor prognosis.
    d) Staging studies for pediatric lymphomas should include an MRI scan of the brain.

The correct answer is (**b**). Lymphoma that is early PET responsive has an excellent prognosis; however, persistent FDG uptake after front-line chemotherapy is considered a relapse. Lymphoma is the most common anterior mediastinal mass in children. Staging for pediatric lymphoma should include a chest X-ray as well as chest, abdomen, and pelvic CT scans; however, brain imaging is not typically done unless the patient has neurologic symptoms.

Case 56

1. Which of the following is more common in ulcerative colitis than in Crohn disease?
    a) Sclerosing cholangitis
    b) Skip lesions
    c) Fistulas
    d) Perianal disease

The correct answer is (**a**). Skip lesions, fistulas, and perianal disease are more common in Crohn disease than in ulcerative colitis. By contrast, sclerosing cholangitis is much more frequently associated with ulcerative colitis.

2. Which part of the bowel is most frequently involved in Crohn disease?
    a) Duodenum
    b) Jejunum
    c) Ileum
    d) Colon

The correct answer is (**c**). Although Crohn disease can involve any part of the alimentary canal, it most commonly affects the ileum, and the terminal ileum in particular, which is involved in more than 9 out of 10 patients.

Case 57

1. Which of the following does not represent a potential site of an apophyseal injury?
    a) Tibial tubercle
    b) Medial epicondyle of the humerus
    c) Patella
    d) Iliac crest

The correct answer is (**c**). The tibial tubercle, medial epicondyle of the humerus, and iliac crest are all important sites at which apophyseal injuries can occur. The patella, by contrast, does not represent an apophysis.

2. Surgery is generally considered when the displacement associated with an apophyseal avulsion fracture exceeds what length?
   a) 0 cm
   b) 1 cm
   c) 2 cm
   d) 3 cm

The correct answer is (**c**). Even though there is no hard-and-fast rule, when the degree of displacement is < 2 cm, surgery is unlikely to be necessary unless symptoms persist after several months of decreased activity.

■ Case 58
....

1. Infants with anomalous origin of the coronary artery typically present with which of the following?
   a) Cyanosis
   b) Failure to thrive
   c) Syncope
   d) Chest pain

The correct answer is (**b**). Patients with anomalous origin of the left coronary artery have little shunting, which is generally left to right, so there is no cyanosis. Syncope and chest pain are presenting symptoms in older children and adolescents. Nonspecific failure to thrive is a common presentation for infants with this condition.

2. In anomalous origin of the left coronary artery, which is the cardiac chamber with the greatest degree of decreased function?
   a) Right atrium
   b) Right ventricle
   c) Left atrium
   d) Left ventricle

The correct answer is (**d**). Because tissue supplied by the left coronary artery is most severely affected and the left ventricle has the greatest perfusion demands, the left ventricle is the most severely dysfunctional chamber.

■ Case 59
....

1. Which of the following is not associated with asplenia?
   a) Aorta and inferior vena cava on same side
   b) Trilobed lungs
   c) Azygous continuation of the inferior vena cava
   d) Anomalous pulmonary venous connection

The correct answer is (**c**). Ipsilateral aorta and inferior vena cava, trilobed lungs, and anomalous pulmonary venous connection are all associated with asplenia. By contrast, azygous continuation of the inferior vena cava is found in patients with polysplenia.

2. Which of the following imaging modalities is most useful in infants with suspected heterotaxy syndrome?
   a) Ultrasound
   b) CT
   c) MRI
   d) Nuclear medicine

The correct answer is (**a**). In specific situations, CT, MRI, and nuclear medicine may each prove helpful in evaluating a patient with heterotaxy, but echocardiography and abdominal ultrasound are the first-line studies when heterotaxy is suspected.

■ Case 60
....

1. Which is true concerning the presence of follicles on the ovaries?
   a) Is never normal in a newborn
   b) Can be normal at any age
   c) Is only normal after puberty
   d) Indicates that the patient is ovulating

The correct answer is (**b**). After birth, follicle stimulating hormone (FSH) rises in the newborn period. During the 2nd year of life, the FSH level decreases but a low level of pulsatile FSH secretion persists. So, the ovary contains mature follicles at all ages.

2. Congenital unilateral renal agenesis is associated with which condition?
   a) Unilateral testicular agenesis
   b) Micropenis
   c) Early menarche
   d) Unicornuate uterus

The correct answer is (**d**). Genital anomalies occur in up to 60% of females and 12% of males with congenital unilateral renal agenesis. In females, a multitude of anomalies of the uterus, ovaries, and vagina can occur. In males, the abnormalities include cryptorchidism, seminal vesicle cysts, hypoplastic vas, unilateral prostatic agenesis, cystic testicular dysplasia, and hypospadias.

Case 61

1. Which of the following is not an important risk factor for the development of pseudomembranous colitis?
   a) Immunosuppression
   b) Antibiotic use
   c) Past history of pseudomembranous colitis
   d) Age < 1 year

The correct answer is (**d**). Immunosuppression, antibiotic use, and a past history of the disorder all increase the risk of developing pseudomembranous colitis. By contrast, the disorder is rare in patients < 1 year of age.

2. On abdominal radiographs, thumbprinting is usually most pronounced in what part of the colon?
   a) Cecum
   b) Transverse colon
   c) Descending colon
   d) Sigmoid colon

The correct answer is (**b**). Because the transverse colon is the most ventral or anterior of these structures, bowel gas tends to collect here in a supine patient, which makes thumbprinting most apparent in this part of the colon.

Case 62

1. Which of the following is the most likely etiology of ileal atresia?
   a) Failure of recanalization
   b) In utero vascular accident
   c) Volvulus
   d) Inspissated meconium

The correct answer is (**b**). Failure of recanalization is the likely etiology of duodenal atresia. Volvulus can cause atresia, but it is not believed to be the cause in most cases. Inspissated meconium may also cause atresia but is most closely associated with meconium ileus. Most cases of ileal atresia are thought to result from in utero vascular accidents.

2. What condition is most likely to be associated with ileal atresia?
   a) Gastroschisis
   b) Duodenal atresia
   c) Meconium plug syndrome
   d) Hirschsprung disease

The correct answer is (**a**). Duodenal atresia occurs by a different mechanism and has no strong association with ileal atresia. Meconium plug syndrome is not associated with atresias. Likewise, Hirschsprung disease occurs by a different mechanism and has no particular association with ileal atresia. By contrast, gastroschisis, in which the bowel is suspended outside the abdomen and unprotected from amniotic fluid, has a relatively strong association with ileal atresia.

Case 63

1. In patients with supracondylar fractures, pulselessness of the hand is most commonly associated with compromise of which artery?
   a) Radial artery
   b) Ulnar artery
   c) Axillary artery
   d) Brachial artery

The correct answer is (**d**). The brachial artery is the vessel most commonly compromised in patients with a supracondylar fracture and pulseless hand. Forms of injury include entrapment, laceration, and spasm.

2. Which of the following is not an important complication of displaced supracondylar fractures?
   a) Neurovascular injury
   b) Intra-articular loose body
   c) Cubitus varus
   d) Avascular necrosis

The answer is (**c**). Neurovascular injury, intra-articular loose body, and avascular necrosis are all associated with functional impairment of the elbow. Cubitus varus, also known as gunstock deformity, can result from supracondylar fractures but is not associated with limitation of motion.

Case 64

1. What is the most common location of venolymphatic malformations?
   a) Abdomen
   b) Thorax
   c) Extremities
   d) Head and neck

The correct answer is (**d**). Nearly half of venolymphatic malformations are located in the head and neck.

2. Which of the following lesions exhibits the least blood flow?
   a) Arteriovenous malformation
   b) Infantile hemangioma
   c) Venous malformation
   d) Lymphatic malformation

Case 72

1. In which of the following disorders do patients typically present with thrombocytopenia?
   a) Henoch–Schönlein purpura
   b) Ulcerative colitis
   c) Hemolytic-uremic syndrome
   d) Crohn disease

The correct answer is (**c**). Reduced platelet levels are a characteristic feature of hemolytic-uremic syndrome (disseminated intravascular thrombosis), whereas platelet levels in Henoch–Schönlein purpura are generally normal or increased.

2. In Henoch–Schönlein purpura, in which part of the intestine are hemorrhage and edema typically most prominent?
   a) Duodenum
   b) Jejunum
   c) Ileum
   d) Colon

The correct answer is (**b**). The jejunum is the most common site of gastrointestinal hemorrhage in Henoch–Schönlein purpura.

Case 73

1. Which of the following constitutes the most important contraindication to contrast enema in a newborn with suspected distal bowel obstruction?
   a) Failure to pass meconium
   b) Abdominal distention
   c) Pneumoperitoneum
   d) Bilious vomiting

The correction answer is (**c**). Failure to pass meconium, abdominal distention, and bilious vomiting are all indications for a contrast enema, although bilious vomiting should also raise suspicion for malrotation with midgut volvulus, and a barium upper GI examination should also be considered. By contrast, pneumoperitoneum indicates a bowel perforation, necessitating surgical intervention. Infusing contrast material into the bowel would only increase the probability of peritonitis and sepsis.

2. Which of the following is not a complication of Hirschsprung disease?
   a) Fistula formation
   b) Toxic megacolon
   c) Perforation
   d) Sepsis

The correct answer is (**a**). With chronic obstruction, toxic megacolon may result, which can lead to both perforation and sepsis. By contrast, chronic inflammation of the colon in Hirschsprung disease is generally not transmural and therefore does not tend to result in fistula formation.

Case 74

1. Which of the following imaging findings is most specific for splenic laceration?
   a) Subcapsular hematoma
   b) Elevated left hemidiaphragm
   c) Left pleural effusion
   d) Left rib fracture

The correct answer is (**a**). Elevated left hemidiaphragm, left pleural effusion, and left rib fracture are all associated with splenic injury, but each can be present for other reasons. By contrast, a subcapsular hematoma is relatively specific for splenic injury.

2. Which is most helpful in determining whether a patient with a splenic laceration can be managed without surgery?
   a) Depth of laceration in the splenic parenchyma
   b) Size of subcapsular hematoma
   c) Density of perisplenic fluid collection
   d) Hemodynamic instability

The correct answer is (**d**). The morphology and associated fluid collections in splenic laceration are less important in assessing the need for operative management than whether or not the patient is hemodynamically unstable.

Case 75

1. The abnormal appearance of which structure in the brain gives rise to the molar tooth sign?
   a) Corpus callosum
   b) Inferior cerebellar peduncles
   c) Cerebellar vermis
   d) Superior cerebellar peduncles

The correct answer is (**d**). The molar tooth appearance results from a lack of normal decussation of superior cerebellar peduncular fiber tracts. This leads to enlargement and a more horizontal course of these tracts.

2. The absence of which structure creates a midline cleft between the cerebellar hemispheres, leading to the batwing appearance of the fourth ventricle on axial images?
    a) Vermis
    b) Superior cerebellar peduncles
    c) Flocculus of the cerebellum
    d) Gracile tubercle

The correct answer is (**a**). The batwing appearance of the fourth ventricle on transverse CT and MR images of the brain is caused by absence of the vermis.

◾ Case 76

1. Which of the following should not raise clinical suspicion for neutropenic colitis in a patient with neutropenia?
    a) Hematemesis
    b) Abdominal pain
    c) Palpable right lower quadrant mass
    d) Fever

The correct answer is (**a**). In a patient with neutropenia, fever, abdominal pain, and palpable right lower quadrant mass are all suggestive of neutropenic colitis. By contrast, hematemesis is not a presenting system of this disorder.

2. Which of the following is not a component of the treatment of neutropenic colitis?
    a) Reduction of immunosuppression
    b) Antiviral medications
    c) Broad-spectrum antibiotics
    d) Bowel rest

The correct answer is (**b**). Restoring neutrophil count to normal, broad-spectrum antibiotics, and bowel rest are all key components of the treatment of neutropenic colitis. By contrast, viruses are not thought to be responsible, and antiviral therapy does not play a role.

◾ Case 77

1. Which of the following types of tracheoesophageal anomaly is most common?
    a) Esophageal atresia without tracheoesophageal fistula
    b) Tracheoesophageal fistula without esophageal atresia
    c) Esophageal atresia with tracheoesophageal fistula
    d) Esophageal atresia with proximal and distal tracheoesophageal fistulas

The correct answer is (**c**). Esophageal atresia with tracheoesophageal fistula constitutes ~85% of tracheoesophageal anomalies.

2. Which of the following radiologic examinations is not indicated when a patient is diagnosed with a tracheoesophageal anomaly?
    a) Renal ultrasound
    b) Echocardiography
    c) Spine radiographs
    d) Barium enema

The correct answer is (**d**). Renal, cardiac, and vertebral anomalies are all components of the VACTERL association. Although anal anomalies are also part of this association, the diagnosis of imperforate anus is established on physical examination, and an enema is not indicated.

◾ Case 78

1. Coarctation of the aorta is most strongly associated with which of the following conditions?
    a) Marfan syndrome
    b) Turner syndrome
    c) Ivemark syndrome
    d) Hypogenetic lung syndrome

The correct answer is (**b**). Approximately one third of patients with Turner syndrome have coarctation of the aorta. Marfan syndrome is associated with aortic aneurysm. Ivemark syndrome is another name for heterotaxy. Hypogenetic lung syndrome is another name for scimitar syndrome.

2. Which of the following is not a common treatment for coarctation of the aorta?
    a) Aortic bypass
    b) Resection with end-to-end anastomosis
    c) Balloon angioplasty
    d) Interposition graft

The correct answer is (**a**). Resection with end-to-end anastomosis, balloon angioplasty, and interposition graft are all common treatments, but aortic bypass is not.

◾ Case 79

1. Which of the following is not a common location of a soft tissue foreign body?
    a) Plantar surface of foot
    b) Anterior aspect of knee
    c) Palmar surface of hand
    d) Posterior surface of neck

The correct answer is (**d**). The plantar surface of the foot, anterior aspect of the knee, and palmar surface of the hand are all common locations of soft tissue foreign bodies, but the neck is not.

2. Which of the following is the most common presentation of a soft tissue foreign body?
   a) Painful mass
   b) Painless mass
   c) Draining wound
   d) Abscess

The correct answer is (**b**). While any of the listed presentations is possible, most soft tissue foreign bodies—particularly those that have been present for weeks or longer—present as painless and often firm soft tissue masses.

■ Case 80

1. Which of the following is the most frequent complication of a simple ovarian cyst in a neonate?
   a) Hemorrhage
   b) Ovarian torsion
   c) Neoplastic transformation
   d) Compression of a ureter leading to hydronephrosis

The correct answer is (**b**). The most frequent complication of a simple ovarian cyst is torsion of the ovary. Cysts > 5 cm should be closely monitored or referred for surgical consultation. Intracystic hemorrhage; cyst rupture; and pressure on nearby structures such as blood vessels, uterus, intestines and urinary system can also occur.

2. A complex ovarian cyst in the newborn is thought to be a result of which of the following?
   a) In utero torsion
   b) Malignant transformation
   c) Rupture
   d) Endometriosis

The correct answer is (**a**). Complex ovarian cysts are thought to be the result of in utero torsion. A complex cyst may require surgical management.

■ Case 81

1. Which of the following is the most common cause of bowel obstruction in young pediatric patients?
   a) Adhesions
   b) Hernias
   c) Volvulus
   d) Intussusception

The correct answer is (**d**). Although adhesions, hernias, volvulus, and intussusception are all relatively common causes of bowel obstruction in young pediatric patients, intussusception is the most common.

2. Which of the following imaging findings is not associated with a decreased probability of radiologic intussusception reduction?
   a) Intussusception in the distal colon
   b) Long duration of symptoms (> 48 hours)
   c) High-grade small-bowel obstruction
   d) Toxic-appearing, lethargic patient

The correct answer is (**a**). Long duration of symptoms, high-grade small-bowel obstruction, and a toxic-appearing, lethargic patient all suggest a decreased probability of successful reduction, whereas the location of the intussusception alone is not associated with a decreased success rate.

■ Case 82

1. Which of the following characteristics of a solid right upper quadrant mass is most important in providing an accurate differential diagnosis?
   a) Degree of enhancement
   b) Organ of origin
   c) Size
   d) Calcification

The correct answer is (**b**). Although degree of enhancement, size, and calcification can be helpful, the most important characteristic among these choices is organ of origin.

2. Which site is the most important to image in the staging of hepatoblastoma?
   a) Lung
   b) Cortical bone
   c) Bone marrow
   d) Brain

The correct answer is (**a**). Hepatoblastoma rarely metastasizes to organs other than the lung.

■ Case 83

1. Which of the following fracture sites is least specific for child abuse?
   a) Clavicle
   b) Sternum
   c) Scapula
   d) Spinous process

The correct answer is (**a**). Fractures of the sternum, scapula, and spinous process are all highly specific for abuse, but clavicle fractures have low specificity.

2. Who is the most common perpetrator of child abuse?
   a) Sibling
   b) Acquaintance
   c) Parent
   d) Stranger

The correct answer is (**c**). In approximately four fifths of cases of child abuse, the perpetrator is a parent.

■ Case 84
....

1. Complications of hepatic laceration in blunt abdominal trauma include each of the following except…
   a) Hepatic infarction
   b) Abscess
   c) Biloma
   d) Delayed hemorrhage

The correct answer is (**b**). Hepatic infarction, biloma, and delayed hemorrhage are all well-known complications of hepatic laceration, but abscess is not a common complication of hepatic laceration in blunt abdominal trauma.

2. What is the best indication for nuclear medicine imaging after liver laceration?
   a) Suspected hepatic infarction
   b) Suspected pseudoaneurysm
   c) Suspected bile leak
   d) Suspected arteriovenous fistula

The correct answer is (**c**). Hepatic infarction, pseudoaneurysm, and arteriovenous fistula are better diagnosed by CT than nuclear medicine. However, a nuclear medicine hepatobiliary examination can be very helpful in detecting extravasation of radiotracer, which establishes the diagnosis of a bile leak.

■ Case 85
....

1. The male urethra is anatomically divided into segments. From proximal to distal, name these segments.
   a) Prostatic, membranous, bulbar, penile
   b) Urogenital, bulbar, membranous, penile
   c) Neck, prostatic, verumontanous, penile
   d) Prostatic, pendulous, penile, fossa navicularis

The correct answer is (**a**). The prostatic urethra is ~3 cm long and is surrounded by the prostate gland. The membranous urethra is 1 cm long and passes through the urogenital diaphragm. The bulbous urethra traverses the root of the penis. The penile urethra is the longest portion. The fossa navicularis refers to the small, normal dilation of the distal penile urethra. The verumontanum is a protrusion on the posterior wall of the prostatic urethra where the seminal ducts enter.

2. The keyhole sign in posterior urethral valves is caused by dilation of what structure?
   a) Base of the bladder
   b) Prostatic urethra
   c) Bulbous urethra
   d) The utricle of the urethra

The correct answer is (**b**). Dilation of the prostatic urethra causes the keyhole sign. The utricle, which has no function, is a diverticulum of the prostatic urethra. It is the male equivalent of the female uterus and vagina.

■ Case 86
....

1. Which of the following is the most common congenital cardiac anomaly?
   a) Atrial septal defect
   b) Ventricular septal defect
   c) Patent ductus arteriosus
   d) Atrioventricular canal

The correct answer is (**b**). Ventricular septal defects are the most common congenital cardiac anomaly and the type most likely to be found in association with other congenital cardiac anomalies.

2. Which of the following congenital cardiac anomalies is always associated with a ventricular septal defect?
   a) Tetralogy of Fallot
   b) Coarctation of the aorta
   c) Tricuspid atresia
   d) Atrial septal defect

The correct answer is (**a**). Tetralogy of Fallot consists of pulmonary stenosis, ventricular septal defect, overriding aorta, and right ventricular hypertrophy. Coarctation of the aorta and tricuspid atresia are associated with ventricular septal defect, although one is not always present. Atrial septal defect does not have a strong association with ventricular septal defect.

■ Case 87

1. On radiographs of premature infants with necrotizing enterocolitis, which of the following is not a sign of pneumoperitoneum?
    a) Triangles of lucency just beneath the abdominal wall on cross-table lateral radiographs
    b) Ovoid and curvilinear lucencies in the bowel wall
    c) Outlining of the falciform ligament by gas
    d) Increasing lucency over the liver

The correct answer is (**b**). Triangles of lucency, visualization of the falciform ligament, and increased lucency over the liver are all classic findings of pneumoperitoneum. Ovoid and curvilinear lucencies in the bowel wall represent the typical appearance of pneumatosis intestinalis, not pneumoperitoneum.

2. Which of the following is not a serious complication of necrotizing enterocolitis?
    a) Portal venous gas
    b) Bowel perforation
    c) Bowel stricture
    d) Short gut syndrome

The correct answer is (**a**). Bowel perforation, delayed development of bowel stricture, and short gut syndrome secondary to bowel ischemia and infarction are all serious complications of necrotizing enterocolitis. Portal venous gas is a radiographic finding that strongly supports the diagnosis but does not by itself represent a serious threat to health or life.

■ Case 88

1. Which of the following clinical presentations is most consistent with duodenal atresia?
    a) Inability to pass an orogastric tube
    b) Bilious vomiting
    c) Choking with feeds
    d) Failure to pass meconium

The correct answer is (**b**). Difficulty passing an orogastric tube and choking with feeds are most characteristic of esophageal atresia. Failure to pass meconium is more typical of a distal bowel obstruction, such as Hirschsprung disease or meconium plug syndrome. Bilious vomiting is a common presentation of duodenal atresia, although depending on the level at which the duodenum is obstructed, the vomitus need not contain bile.

2. On an abdominal radiograph, which of the following conditions is most commonly associated with a triple bubble?
    a) Hypertrophic pyloric stenosis
    b) Jejunal atresia
    c) Ileal atresia
    d) Colonic atresia

The correct answer is (**b**). In hypertrophic pyloric stenosis, the gastric outlet is obstructed, so there is typically only one bubble. In ileal and colonic atresia, the obstruction is distal, so there are many segments of dilated bowel. In proximal jejunal atresia, there are often three bubbles: dilated stomach, dilated duodenum, and dilated proximal jejunum.

■ Case 89

1. Approximately how many radiographic views are recommended by the American Academy of Pediatrics in a skeletal survey to evaluate suspected child abuse?
    a) 6
    b) 12
    c) 18
    d) 22

The correct answer is (**d**). Recommended views include anteroposterior (AP) views of both arms, both forearms, both hands, both thighs, both legs, both feet, thorax AP and lateral, AP abdomen, AP lumbar spine, AP bony pelvis, lateral lumbar spine, AP and lateral cervical spine, and frontal and lateral skull.

2. Which of the following is not a condition that predisposes infants to skeletal fractures?
    a) Osteogenesis imperfecta
    b) Spondylometaphyseal dysplasia
    c) Menkes syndrome
    d) Rickets

The correct answer is (**b**). Osteogenesis imperfecta, Menkes syndrome, and rickets are all associated with bone fragility and increased probability of fracture. In spondylometaphyseal dysplasia, metaphyseal irregularities may resemble corner fractures but generally do not in fact represent fractures.

▣ Case 90

1. A 1-year-old boy presents with a large renal mass. Upon further imaging, a cerebellar astrocytoma was discovered. The renal tumor is most likely which of the following?
    a) Rhabdoid tumor
    b) Angiomyolipoma
    c) Wilms tumor
    d) Clear cell sarcoma

The correct answer is (**a**). Association with primitive neuroectodermal tumor, ependymoma, and cerebellar and brainstem astrocytoma as well as early brain metastases is highly distinctive of rhabdoid tumors.

2. Which of the following tumors is not associated with invasion of the renal vein?
    a) Rhabdoid tumor
    b) Wilms tumor
    c) Renal medullary carcinoma
    d) Clear cell sarcoma

The correct answer is (**d**). Wilms tumor, renal medullary carcinoma, and rhabdoid tumor all invade the renal vein. Clear cell sarcoma is generally not associated with vascular invasion.

▣ Case 91

1. Which of the following is not a complication of Langerhans cell histiocytosis?
    a) Pathologic fracture
    b) Diabetes insipidus
    c) Anemia
    d) Mental retardation

The correct answer is (**d**). Pathologic fracture, diabetes insipidus (due to involvement of the pituitary stalk), and anemia (a poor prognostic sign) are all complications of Langerhans cell histiocytosis. Mental retardation is not.

2. Bone lesions in Langerhans cell histiocytosis can appear as which of the following?
    a) Lytic
    b) Sclerotic
    c) Poorly defined
    d) All of the above

The correct answer is (**d**). Although most lesions in Langerhans cell histiocytosis are lytic, they can appear lytic or sclerotic, and well-defined or poorly defined, and they may or may not exhibit periosteal reaction.

▣ Case 92

1. Which of the following would not increase the probability of meconium ileus in a neonate who presents with a bowel obstruction?
    a) The patient has a sibling with cystic fibrosis.
    b) Passage of meconium occurs within 24 hours of birth.
    c) The patient is Caucasian.
    d) Prenatal ultrasound showed peritoneal calcifications.

The correct answer is (**b**). Meconium ileus is highly associated with cystic fibrosis, an autosomally recessive condition, so having a sibling with cystic fibrosis would increase the probability of cystic fibrosis, as opposed to a patient with no family history of the disorder. Cystic fibrosis is far less likely among non-Caucasians. The prenatal ultrasound finding of peritoneal calcifications suggests an in utero bowel perforation, which is associated with meconium ileus. Spontaneous passage of meconium within 24 hours of birth would essentially rule out the diagnosis of meconium ileus.

2. Which of the following diagnoses should not be suspected in a patient found to have a total microcolon on contrast enema?
    a) Megacystis-microcolon-hypoperistalsis syndrome
    b) Ileal atresia
    c) Meconium ileus
    d) Duodenal atresia

The correct answer is (**d**). As the name implies, megacystis-microcolon-hypoperistalsis syndrome is associated with microcolon, as are ileal atresia and meconium ileus, both of which involve distal small bowel obstruction. By contrast, duodenal atresia is a proximal obstruction, which allows a sufficient amount of bowel contents from small bowel distal to the obstruction to reach the colon to prevent a microcolon.

▣ Case 93

1. Which of the following is not a common presenting complaint in patients diagnosed with gastrointestinal duplication cysts?
    a) Abdominal mass
    b) Vomiting
    c) Hematemesis
    d) Asymptomatic

The correct answer is (**c**). Relatively common presentations of patients with gastrointestinal duplication cysts include incidental discovery in asymptomatic patients, abdominal mass, and vomiting (due to obstruction). By contrast, although such cysts may hemorrhage, hematemesis is quite uncommon.

2. Which of the following is not a complication of
   gastrointestinal duplication cysts?
   a) Malignant transformation
   b) Perforation
   c) Intussusception
   d) Bowel obstruction

The correct answer is (**a**). Perforation, intussusception
(with the duplication cyst acting as lead point), and bowel
obstruction have all been reported as complications of
duplication cysts. However, malignant transformation is not
a complication because these lesions are not neoplasms.

■ Case 94
....

1. In an infant with a liver mass, what physical
   clinical finding is most specific for infantile
   hemangioendothelioma?
   a) Large size of mass
   b) Abdominal distention
   c) Bruit over mass
   d) Female patient

The correct answer is (**c**). Patients with infantile
hemangioendothelioma may have a larger mass and
abdominal distention, but neither of these findings is
very specific. Likewise, infantile hemangioendothelioma
is more common in girls, but only slightly so. By contrast,
a bruit over the mass is strongly suggestive of vascular
shunting, which is relatively specific for infantile
hemangioendothelioma.

2. What is the most common cause of death in patients
   with infantile hemangioendothelioma?
   a) Congestive heart failure
   b) Mass effect on adjacent organs
   c) Malignant transformation to sarcoma
   d) Complications of corticosteroid therapy

The correct answer is (**a**). Large infantile
hemangioendotheliomas can exert considerable mass
effect on adjacent organs, sarcomatous transformation has
been reported in rare cases, and corticosteroids are often
used in the treatment of symptomatic lesions. However,
the most common cause of death in patients with infantile
hemangioendothelioma is congestive heart failure.

■ Case 95
....

1. What is the most common location for a nonmidline
   thyroglossal duct cyst?
   a) At the base of the tongue
   b) At the level of the hyoid bone
   c) Next to the cricoid cartilage
   d) Next to the thyroid cartilage

The correct answer is (**d**). When thyroglossal duct cysts are
located off midline, they are usually tucked next to the thyroid cartilage. Of note, the more inferior the lesion is, the
more likely it is to be off midline.

2. What is the most common neck mass in a child?
   a) Thyroglossal duct cyst
   b) Branchial cleft cyst
   c) Lymphadenopathy
   d) Cystic hygroma

The correct answer is (**c**). Lymphadenopathy is the most
common neck mass in a child. It is much more common
than a thyroglossal duct cyst, which is the most common
congenital neck mass in a child. Thyroglossal duct cysts are
~3 times more common than branchial cleft cysts.

■ Case 96
....

1. Which of the following is an unusual setting for a tibial
   stress injury?
   a) Recent military recruit
   b) Athlete
   c) Previously sedentary teen who took up jogging
   d) Patient who heard a "pop" and suffered sudden-
      onset shin pain

The correct answer is (**d**). By definition, stress injuries
do not present with a distinct episode of trauma or a
sudden onset of symptoms. Military recruits, athletes,
and individuals who increase their level of activity are
all common settings for stress injuries.

2. Once the cast is removed from patients who have been
   casted for a tibial stress injury, such patients are at
   increased risk for which of the following?
   a) Osteomyelitis
   b) Ewing sarcoma
   c) Insufficiency fracture
   d) Osteoid osteoma

The correct answer is (**c**). Decreased use and hyperemia
associated with healing can both promote the development
of osteopenia, which places the patient at increased risk for
insufficiency fracture upon return to normal activity.

■ Case 97
....

1. After chest radiograph, which should be the initial
   imaging modality for most patients with suspected
   anomalous venous connection?
   a) Echocardiography
   b) CT
   c) MRI
   d) Nuclear medicine

The correct answer is (**a**). Echocardiography is the initial imaging study of choice in virtually all forms of congenital heart disease, including anomalous pulmonary venous connection.

2. Which of the following is not a disadvantage of MRI, as compared to CT, in the postoperative evaluation of a patient with total anomalous pulmonary venous connection?
    a) Long image acquisition time
    b) Frequent need for sedation
    c) Susceptibility to metal artifact
    d) Multiplanar imaging

The correct answer is (**d**). Long image acquisition time, frequent need for sedation, and metal susceptibility are all disadvantages of MRI, whereas multiplanar imaging is an advantage of MRI.

Case 98

1. In general, which is the most appropriate first imaging examination in a pediatric patient with suspected acute appendicitis?
    a) Abdominal radiograph
    b) CT of the abdomen and pelvis
    c) Ultrasound of the right lower quadrant
    d) Barium enema

The correct answer is (**c**). If the specificity of clinical findings is low and other etiologies such as bowel obstruction are also under consideration, plain radiographs may be an appropriate first imaging alternative. Likewise, if other etiologies are equally likely, there is high clinical suspicion of perforation, or there is little local experience with right lower quadrant ultrasound, CT may be more appropriate. Barium enema currently plays no role the evaluation of appendicitis. If appendicitis is at the top of the differential diagnosis, the patient is not obese, and the exam will be performed by an experienced sonographer, ultrasound is both a highly accurate examination and reduces radiation exposure and cost.

2. Important mimics of acute appendicitis include each of the following except…
    a) Mesenteric adenitis
    b) Ovarian torsion
    c) Omental infarction
    d) Diverticulitis

The correct answer is (**d**). Mesenteric adenitis, ovarian torsion, and omental infarction are all important mimics of appendicitis. By contrast, diverticulitis is relatively uncommon in the pediatric population and more commonly presents with pain in the left lower quadrant.

Case 99

1. Which part of the bowel is most commonly injured in blunt abdominal trauma?
    a) Duodenum
    b) Ileum
    c) Colon
    d) Rectum

The correct answer is (**a**). Although any part of the bowel may be injured in blunt abdominal trauma, the duodenum is the most common site of these choices, perhaps because it is often pinched between the anterior abdominal wall and the spine.

2. Which of the following findings represents the strongest indication for surgery in a patient who suffered blunt abdominal trauma?
    a) Ascites
    b) Bowel wall thickening
    c) Pneumoperitoneum
    d) Abnormally intense bowel wall enhancement

The correct answer is (**c**). Ascites, bowel wall thickening, and abnormally intense bowel wall enhancement can all be signs of bowel injury, but pneumoperitoneum is the only one that indicates perforation, for which surgery is indicated.

Case 100

1. Which of the following is the most commonly diagnosed lung anomaly in the prenatal period?
    a) Congenital pulmonary airway malformation
    b) Bronchogenic cyst
    c) Pulmonary sequestration
    d) Bronchial atresia

The correct answer is (**a**). Congenital pulmonary airway malformation is the most common prenatally diagnosed lung malformation and constitutes approximately one quarter of congenital lung malformations. Each of the others is less commonly diagnosed in the prenatal period.

2. In which lobe is congenital pulmonary airway malformation least frequently seen?
    a) Upper lobe
    b) Middle lobe
    c) Lower lobe

The correct answer is (**b**). Congenital pulmonary airway malformations are rarely found in the middle lobe. When present there, they normally communicate with the tracheobronchial tree.

Further Readings

■ Case 1

Lampl B, Levin TL, Berdon WE, Cowles RA. Malrotation and midgut volvulus: a historical review and current controversies in diagnosis and management. Pediatr Radiol 2009;39(4):359–366

Laurence N, Pollock AN. Malrotation with midgut volvulus. Pediatr Emerg Care 2012;28(1):87–89

Shew SB. Surgical concerns in malrotation and midgut volvulus. Pediatr Radiol 2009;39(Suppl 2):S167–S171

■ Case 2

Agarwal R. Prenatal diagnosis of anterior abdominal wall defects: pictorial essay. Indian J Radiol Imaging 2005;15(3):361–372

Daltro P, Fricke BL, Kline-Fath BM, et al. Prenatal MRI of congenital abdominal and chest wall defects. AJR Am J Roentgenol 2005;184(3):1010–1016

■ Case 3

Aksoy Ozcan U, Altun E, Abbasoglu L. Space occupying lesions in the fetal chest evaluated by MRI. Iran J Radiol 2012;9(3):122–129

Daltro P, Werner H, Gasparetto TD, et al. Congenital chest malformations: a multimodality approach with emphasis on fetal MR imaging. Radiographics 2010;30(2):385–395

Liu YP, Chen CP, Shih SL, Chen YF, Yang FS, Chen SC. Fetal cystic lung lesions: evaluation with magnetic resonance imaging. Pediatr Pulmonol 2010;45(6):592–600

Mehollin-Ray AR, Cassady CI, Cass DL, Olutoye OO. Fetal MR imaging of congenital diaphragmatic hernia. Radiographics 2012;32(4):1067–1084

■ Case 4

Chao TT, Dashe JS, Adams RC, Keefover-Hicks A, McIntire DD, Twickler DM. Fetal spine findings on MRI and associated outcomes in children with open neural tube defects. AJR Am J Roentgenol 2011;197(5):W956–W961

Geerdink N, van der Vliet T, Rotteveel JJ, Feuth T, Roeleveld N, Mullaart RA. Essential features of Chiari II malformation in MR imaging: an interobserver reliability study—part 1. Childs Nerv Syst 2012;28(7):977–985

Mangels KJ, Tulipan N, Tsao LY, Alarcon J, Bruner JP. Fetal MRI in the evaluation of intrauterine myelomeningocele. Pediatr Neurosurg 2000;32(3):124–131

Mirsky DM, Schwartz ES, Zarnow DM. Diagnostic features of myelomeningocele: the role of ultrafast fetal MRI. Fetal Diagn Ther 2015;37(3):219–225

■ Case 5

Agarwal R, Khan A, Garg M, Aggarwal AN, Gupta D. Pictorial essay: allergic bronchopulmonary aspergillosis. Indian J Radiol Imaging 2011;21(4):242–252

Franquet T, Müller NL, Giménez A, Guembe P, de La Torre J, Bagué S. Spectrum of pulmonary aspergillosis: histologic, clinical, and radiologic findings. Radiographics 2001;21(4):825–837

■ Case 6

Brody JM, Leighton DB, Murphy BL, et al. CT of blunt trauma bowel and mesenteric injury: typical findings and pitfalls in diagnosis. Radiographics 2000;20(6):1525–1536, discussion 1536–1537

Daly KP, Ho CP, Persson DL, Gay SB. Traumatic retroperitoneal injuries: review of multidetector CT findings. Radiographics 2008;28(6):1571–1590

Linsenmaier U, Wirth S, Reiser M, Körner M. Diagnosis and classification of pancreatic and duodenal injuries in emergency radiology. Radiographics 2008;28(6): 1591–1602

■ Case 7

Gun F, Erginel B, Unüvar A, Kebudi R, Salman T, Celik A. Mediastinal masses in children: experience with 120 cases. Pediatr Hematol Oncol 2012;29(2):141–147

Patel IJ, Hsiao E, Ahmad AH, Schroeder C, Gilkeson RC. AIRP best cases in radiologic-pathologic correlation: mediastinal mature cystic teratoma. Radiographics 2013;33(3):797–801

Ranganath SH, Lee EY, Restrepo R, Eisenberg RL.
    Mediastinal masses in children. AJR Am J Roentgenol
    2012;198(3):W197–W216

■ Case 8

Berrocal T, López-Pereira P, Arjonilla A, Gutiérrez J.
    Anomalies of the distal ureter, bladder, and urethra
    in children: embryologic, radiologic, and pathologic
    features. Radiographics 2002;22(5):1139–1164

Cruz-Diaz O, Salomon A, Rosenberg E, et al. Anterior
    urethral valves: not such a benign condition. . . .
    Front Pediatr 2013;1:35

Levin TL, Han B, Little BP. Congenital anomalies of the male
    urethra. Pediatr Radiol 2007;37(9):851–862, quiz 945

■ Case 9

Koeller KK, Rosenblum RS, Morrison AL. Neoplasms of the
    spinal cord and filum terminale: radiologic-pathologic
    correlation. Radiographics 2000;20(6):1721–1749

Seo HS, Kim JH, Lee DH, et al. Nonenhancing
    intramedullary astrocytomas and other MR imaging
    features: a retrospective study and systematic review.
    AJNR Am J Neuroradiol 2010;31(3):498–503

■ Case 10

Koeller KK, Alamo L, Adair CF, Smirniotopoulos JG.
    Congenital cystic masses of the neck: radiologic-
    pathologic correlation. Radiographics 1999;19(1):
    121–146, quiz 152–153

Lanham PD, Wushensky C. Second brachial cleft
    cyst mimic: case report. AJNR Am J Neuroradiol
    2005;26(7):1862–1864

■ Case 11

Donnelly LF, Frush DP, Marshall KW, White KS.
    Lymphoproliferative disorders: CT findings in
    immunocompromised children. AJR Am J Roentgenol
    1998;171(3):725–731

Pickhardt PJ, Siegel MJ, Hayashi RJ, Kelly M.
    Posttransplantation lymphoproliferative disorder in
    children: clinical, histopathologic, and imaging features.
    Radiology 2000;217(1):16–25

Scarsbrook AF, Warakaulle DR, Dattani M, Traill Z.
    Post-transplantation lymphoproliferative disorder:
    the spectrum of imaging appearances. Clin Radiol
    2005;60(1):47–55

■ Case 12

Bourekas EC, Varakis K, Bruns D, et al. Lesions of
    the corpus callosum: MR imaging and differential
    considerations in adults and children. AJR Am J
    Roentgenol 2002;179(1):251–257

Ho ML, Moonis G, Ginat DT, Eisenberg RL. Lesions of the
    corpus callosum. AJR Am J Roentgenol 2013;200(1):
    W1–W16

Kazi AZ, Joshi PC, Kelkar AB, Mahajan MS, Ghawate AS.
    MRI evaluation of pathologies affecting the corpus
    callosum: A pictorial essay. Indian J Radiol Imaging
    2013;23(4):321–332

■ Case 13

Geerdink N, van der Vliet T, Rotteveel JJ, Feuth T,
    Roeleveld N, Mullaart RA. Essential features of Chiari II
    malformation in MR imaging: an interobserver reliability
    study—part 1. Childs Nerv Syst 2012;28(7):977–985

Hadley DM. The Chiari malformations. J Neurol Neurosurg
    Psychiatry 2002;72(Suppl 2):ii38–ii40

■ Case 14

Rufener SL, Ibrahim M, Raybaud CA, Parmar HA. Congenital
    spine and spinal cord malformations—pictorial review.
    AJR Am J Roentgenol 2010;194(3, Suppl)S26–S37

Sharma P, Kumar S, Jaiswal A. Clinico-radiologic findings
    in group II caudal regression syndrome. J Clin Imaging
    Sci 2013;3:26

■ Case 15

Biyyam DR, Chapman T, Ferguson MR, Deutsch G, Dighe MK.
    Congenital lung abnormalities: embryologic features,
    prenatal diagnosis, and postnatal radiologic-pathologic
    correlation. Radiographics 2010;30(6):1721–1738

Odev K, Guler I, Altinok T, Pekcan S, Batur A, Ozbiner H.
    Cystic and cavitary lung lesions in children: radiologic
    findings with pathologic correlation. J Clin Imaging Sci
    2013;3:60

Paterson A. Imaging evaluation of congenital lung abnormalities in infants and children. Radiol Clin North Am 2005;43(2):303–323

■ Case 16

Arora R, Trehan V, Kumar A, Kalra GS, Nigam M. Transcatheter closure of congenital ventricular septal defects: experience with various devices. J Interv Cardiol 2003;16(1):83–91

Holzer R, Balzer D, Cao Q-L, Lock K, Hijazi ZM; Amplatzer Muscular Ventricular Septal Defect Investigators. Device closure of muscular ventricular septal defects using the Amplatzer muscular ventricular septal defect occluder: immediate and mid-term results of a U.S. registry. J Am Coll Cardiol 2004;43(7):1257–1263

■ Case 17

Aly NT, Towbin AJ, Towbin RB. Pediatric radiological case: diastematomyelia. Appl Radiol 2014;Aug 21

Cheng B, Li FT, Lin L. Diastematomyelia: a retrospective review of 138 patients. J Bone Joint Surg Br 2012;94(3):365–372

Rufener SL, Ibrahim M, Raybaud CA, Parmar HA. Congenital spine and spinal cord malformations—pictorial review. AJR Am J Roentgenol 2010;194(3, Suppl)S26–S37

Unsinn KM, Geley T, Freund MC, Gassner I. US of the spinal cord in newborns: spectrum of normal findings, variants, congenital anomalies, and acquired diseases. Radiographics 2000;20(4):923–938

■ Case 18

Bosemani T, Orman G, Boltshauser E, Tekes A, Huisman TA, Poretti A. Congenital abnormalities of the posterior fossa. Radiographics 2015;35(1):200–220

Epelman M, Daneman A, Blaser SI, et al. Differential diagnosis of intracranial cystic lesions at head US: correlation with CT and MR imaging. Radiographics 2006;26(1):173–196

Shekdar K. Posterior fossa malformations. Semin Ultrasound CT MR 2011;32(3):228–241

■ Case 19

Cerwinka WH, Grattan-Smith JD, Scherz HC, Kirsch AJ. Appearance of Deflux implants with magnetic resonance imaging after endoscopic treatment of vesicoureteral reflux in children. J Pediatr Urol 2009;5(2):114–118

Cerwinka WH, Kaye JD, Scherz HC, Kirsch AJ, Grattan-Smith JD. Radiologic features of implants after endoscopic treatment of vesicoureteral reflux in children. AJR Am J Roentgenol 2010;195(1):234–240

Leopold I, Vollert K, Schuster T. The value of the sonographic appearance of the Deflux deposit following endoscopic VUR-therapy in respect of therapeutic success. J Pediatr Urol 2007;3:S15

■ Case 20

Mermuys K, Jeuris W, Vanhoenacker PK, Van Hoe L, D'Haenens P. Best cases from the AFIP: supratentorial ependymoma. Radiographics 2005;25(2):486–490

Yuh EL, Barkovich AJ, Gupta N. Imaging of ependymomas: MRI and CT. Childs Nerv Syst 2009;25(10):1203–1213

■ Case 21

Furukawa A, Sakoda M, Yamasaki M, et al. Gastrointestinal tract perforation: CT diagnosis of presence, site, and cause. Abdom Imaging 2005;30(5):524–534

Grassi R, Romano S, Pinto A, Romano L. Gastro-duodenal perforations: conventional plain film, US and CT findings in 166 consecutive patients. Eur J Radiol 2004;50(1):30–36

Linsenmaier U, Wirth S, Reiser M, Körner M. Diagnosis and classification of pancreatic and duodenal injuries in emergency radiology. Radiographics 2008;28(6):1591–1602

■ Case 22

Berrocal T, Madrid C, Novo S, Gutiérrez J, Arjonilla A, Gómez-León N. Congenital anomalies of the tracheobronchial tree, lung, and mediastinum: embryology, radiology, and pathology. Radiographics 2004;24(1):e17

Zylak CJ, Eyler WR, Spizarny DL, Stone CH. Developmental lung anomalies in the adult: radiologic-pathologic correlation. Radiographics 2002;22(Spec No, S1)S25–S43

■ Case 23

Chung EM, Cube R, Hall GJ, González C, Stocker JT, Glassman LM. From the archives of the AFIP: breast masses in children and adolescents: radiologic-pathologic correlation. Radiographics 2009;29(3): 907–931

García CJ, Espinoza A, Dinamarca V, et al. Breast US in children and adolescents. Radiographics 2000;20(6):1605–1612

Kaneda HJ, Mack J, Kasales CJ, Schetter S. Pediatric and adolescent breast masses: a review of pathophysiology, imaging, diagnosis, and treatment. AJR Am J Roentgenol 2013;200(2):W204–W212

■ Case 24

Douglas-Akinwande AC, Mourad AA, Pradhan K, Hattab EM. Primary intracranial germinoma presenting as a central skull base lesion. AJNR Am J Neuroradiol 2006;27(2):270–273

Dumrongpisutikul N, Intrapiromkul J, Yousem DM. Distinguishing between germinomas and pineal cell tumors on MR imaging. AJNR Am J Neuroradiol 2012;33(3):550–555

Fang AS, Meyers SP. Magnetic resonance imaging of pineal region tumours. Insights Imaging 2013;4(3):369–382

■ Case 25

Shiota K, Yamada S, Komada M, Ishibashi M. Embryogenesis of holoprosencephaly. Am J Med Genet A 2007;143A(24):3079–3087

Winter TC, Kennedy AM, Woodward PJ. Holoprosencephaly: a survey of the entity, with embryology and fetal imaging. Radiographics 2015;35(1):275–290

■ Case 26

Squarcia U, Macchi C. Transposition of the great arteries. Curr Opin Pediatr 2011;23(5):518–522

Warnes CA. Transposition of the great arteries. Circulation 2006;114(24):2699–2709

■ Case 27

Chaudry G, Perez-Atayde AR, Ngan BY, et al. Imaging of congential mesoblastic nephroma. Pediatr Radiol 2009;39(10):1080–1086

Lowe LH, Isuani BH, Heller RM, et al. Pediatric renal masses: Wilms tumor and beyond. Radiographics 2000;20(6):1585–1603

Sheth MM, Cai G, Goodman TR. AIRP best cases in radiologic-pathologic correlation: congenital mesoblastic nephroma. Radiographics 2012;32(1):99–103

■ Case 28

Aso C, Enríquez G, Fité M, et al. Gray-scale and color Doppler sonography of scrotal disorders in children: an update. Radiographics 2005;25(5):1197–1214

Coursey Moreno C, Small WC, Camacho JC, et al. Testicular tumors: what radiologists need to know—differential diagnosis, staging, and management. Radiographics 2015;35(2):400–415

Ross JH, Kay R. Prepubertal testis tumors. Rev Urol 2004;6(1):11–18

Sung EK, Setty BN, Castro-Aragon I. Sonography of the pediatric scrotum: emphasis on the Ts—torsion, trauma, and tumors. AJR Am J Roentgenol 2012;198(5):996–1003

■ Case 29

O'Brien WT Sr. Neuroimaging manifestations of NF1—a pictorial review. J Am Osteopath Coll Radiol 2015;4(2):16–21

Patel NB, Stacy GS. Musculoskeletal manifestations of neurofibromatosis type 1. AJR Am J Roentgenol 2012;199(1):W99–W106

Rodriguez D, Young Poussaint T. Neuroimaging findings in neurofibromatosis type 1 and 2. Neuroimaging Clin N Am 2004;14(2):149–170, vii

■ Case 30

Hlongwane ST, Pienaar M, Dekker G, et al. Proptosis as a manifestation of neuroblastoma. SA J Radiol 2006;10(4):31–32

Papaioannou G, McHugh K. Neuroblastoma in childhood: review and radiological findings. Cancer Imaging 2005;5(1):116–127

■ Case 31

Applegate KE, Anderson JM, Klatte EC. Intestinal malrotation in children: a problem-solving approach to the upper gastrointestinal series. Radiographics 2006;26(5):1485–1500

Long FR, Kramer SS, Markowitz RI, Taylor GE. Radiographic patterns of intestinal malrotation in children. Radiographics 1996;16(3):547–556, discussion 556–560

Strouse PJ. Disorders of intestinal rotation and fixation ("malrotation"). Pediatr Radiol 2004;34(11):837–851

■ Case 32

Chung EM, Cube R, Hall CJ, et al. Breast masses in children and adolescents: radiologic-pathologic correlation. Radiographics 2009;29:907–931

Garcia CJ, Espinoza A, Dinamarca V, et al. Breast US in children and adolescents. Radiographics 2000;20:1605–1612

Kaneda HJ, Mack J, Kasales CJ, Schetter S. Pediatric and adolescent breast masses: a review of pathophysiology, imaging, diagnosis, and treatment. AJR Am J Roentgenol 2013;200(2):W204–W212

■ Case 33

Chourmouzi D, Papadopoulou E, Konstantinidis M, et al. Manifestations of pilocytic astrocytoma: a pictorial review. Insights Imaging 2014;5(3):387–402

Koeller KK, Rushing EJ. From the archives of the AFIP: pilocytic astrocytoma: radiologic-pathologic correlation. Radiographics 2004;24(6):1693–1708

Panigrahy A, Blüml S. Neuroimaging of pediatric brain tumors: from basic to advanced magnetic resonance imaging (MRI). J Child Neurol 2009;24(11):1343–1365

■ Case 34

Corapçioğlu F, Liman T, Aksu G, et al. A case report with type II pleuropulmonary blastoma: successful treatment with surgery and chemotherapy. Turk J Pediatr 2009;51(1):78–81

Hashemi A, Souzani A, Souzani A, Keshavarzi S. Pleuropulmonary blastoma in children: a case report. Iran J Cancer Prev 2012;5(2):105–107

Zhang H, Xu CW, Wei JG, Zhu GJ, Xu S, Wang J. Infant pleuropulmonary blastoma: report of a rare case and review of literature. Int J Clin Exp Pathol 2015;8(10):13571–13577

■ Case 35

Jeung MY, Gangi A, Gasser B, et al. Imaging of chest wall disorders. Radiographics 1999;19(3):617–637

Samuels TH, Haider MA, Kirkbride P. Poland's syndrome: a mammographic presentation. AJR Am J Roentgenol 1996;166(2):347–348

■ Case 36

Crim JR. Imaging of tarsal coalition. Radiol Clin North Am 2008;46(6):1017–1026, vi

Crim JR, Kjeldsberg KM. Radiographic diagnosis of tarsal coalition. AJR Am J Roentgenol 2004;182(2):323–328

■ Case 37

Kawashima A, Sandler CM, Goldman SM, Raval BK, Fishman EK. CT of renal inflammatory disease. Radiographics 1997;17(4):851–866, discussion 867–868

Seguias L, Srinivasan K, Mehta A. Pediatric renal abscess: a 10-year single-center retrospective analysis. Hosp Pediatr 2012;2(3):161–166

Son J, Lee EY, Restrepo R, Eisenberg RL. Focal renal lesions in pediatric patients. AJR Am J Roentgenol 2012;199(6):W668–W682

■ Case 38

Kalra V, Mirza K, Malhotra A. Plunging ranula. J Radiol Case Rep 2011;5(6):18–24

La'Porte SJ, Juttla JK, Lingam RK, et al. Imaging the floor of the mouth and the sublingual space. Radiographics 2011;31(5):1215–1230

Sheikhi M, Jalalian F, Rashidipoor R, Mosavat F. Plunging ranula of the submandibular area. Dent Res J (Isfahan) 2011;8(Suppl 1):S114–S118

■ Case 39

http://www.aast.org/library/traumatools/injuryscoring
scales.aspx

Chiron P, Hornez E, Boddaert G, et al. Grade IV renal
trauma management. A revision of the AAST renal injury
grading scale is mandatory. Eur J Trauma Emerg Surg
2016;42(2):237–241

Park SJ, Kim JK, Kim KW, Cho KS. MDCT Findings of renal
trauma. AJR Am J Roentgenol 2006;187(2):541–547

Ramchandani P, Buckler PM. Imaging of genitourinary
trauma. AJR Am J Roentgenol 2009;192(6):1514–1523

Srinivasa RN, Akbar SA, Jafri SZ, Howells GA. Genitourinary
trauma: a pictorial essay. Emerg Radiol 2009;16(1):
21–33

■ Case 40

Debnam JM, Guha-Thakurta N. Retropharyngeal and
prevertebral spaces: anatomic imaging and diagnosis.
Otolaryngol Clin North Am 2012;45(6):1293–1310

Hoang JK, Branstetter BF IV, Eastwood JD, Glastonbury
CM. Multiplanar CT and MRI of collections in the
retropharyngeal space: is it an abscess? AJR Am J
Roentgenol 2011;196(4):W426–W432

■ Case 41

Lehmann CL, Arons RR, Loder RT, Vitale MG.
The epidemiology of slipped capital femoral epiphysis:
an update. J Pediatr Orthop 2006;26(3):286–290

Parsons SJ, Barton C, Banerjee R, Kiely NT. Slipped capital
femoral epiphysis. Curr Orthop 2007;21:215–228

■ Case 42

Akpinar E. The tram-track sign: cortical calcifications.
Radiology 2004;231(2):515–516

Cagneaux M, Paoli V, Blanchard G, Ville D, Guibaud L. Pre-
and postnatal imaging of early cerebral damage in Sturge-
Weber syndrome. Pediatr Radiol 2013;43(11):1536–1539

■ Case 43

Bouwman A, Verbeke J, Brand M, et al. Renal medullary
hyperechogenicity in a neonate with oliguria. NDT Plus
2010;3(2):176–178

Daneman A, Navarro OM, Somers GR, Mohanta A, Jarrín JR,
Traubici J. Renal pyramids: focused sonography of
normal and pathologic processes. Radiographics
2010;30(5):1287–1307

Durr-E-Sabih, Khan AN, Craig M, Worrall JA.
Sonographic mimics of renal calculi. J Ultrasound Med
2004;23(10):1361–1367

Pacifici GM. Clinical pharmacology of furosemide in neonates:
a review. Pharmaceuticals (Basel) 2013;6(9):1094–1129

■ Case 44

Aso C, Enríquez G, Fité M, et al. Gray-scale and color
Doppler sonography of scrotal disorders in children:
an update. Radiographics 2005;25(5):1197–1214

Bhatt S, Dogra VS. Role of US in testicular and scrotal
trauma. Radiographics 2008;28(6):1617–1629

Sung EK, Setty BN, Castro-Aragon I. Sonography of the
pediatric scrotum: emphasis on the Ts—torsion, trauma,
and tumors. AJR Am J Roentgenol 2012;198(5):996–1003

■ Case 45

Nasseri F, Eftekhari F. Clinical and radiologic review of
the normal and abnormal thymus: pearls and pitfalls.
Radiographics 2010;30(2):413–428

Nishino M, Ashiku SK, Kocher ON, Thurer RL, Boiselle PM,
Hatabu H. The thymus: a comprehensive review.
Radiographics 2006;26(2):335–348

■ Case 46

Burge D, Drewett M. Meconium plug obstruction. Pediatr
Surg Int 2004;20(2):108–110

Keckler SJ, St Peter SD, Spilde TL, et al. Current
significance of meconium plug syndrome. J Pediatr Surg
2008;43(5):896–898

Krasna IH, Rosenfeld D, Salerno P. Is it necrotizing
enterocolitis, microcolon of prematurity, or delayed
meconium plug? A dilemma in the tiny premature
infant. J Pediatr Surg 1996;31(6):855–858

■ Case 47

Fink KR, Thapa MM, Ishak GE, Pruthi S. Neuroimaging
of pediatric central nervous system cytomegalovirus
infection. Radiographics 2010;30(7):1779–1796

Nickerson JP, Richner B, Santy K, et al. Neuroimaging of pediatric intracranial infection—part 2: TORCH, viral, fungal, and parasitic infections. J Neuroimaging 2012;22(2):e52–e63

■ Case 48

Cleveland RH. A radiologic update on medical diseases of the newborn chest. Pediatr Radiol 1995;25(8):631–637

Guglani L, Lakshminrusimha S, Ryan RM. Transient tachypnea of the newborn. Pediatr Rev 2008;29(11):e59–e65

Wood J, Thomas L. Imaging of neonatal lung disease. J Am Osteopath Coll Radiol 2015;4(1):12–18

■ Case 49

Parada Villavicencio C, Adam SZ, Nikolaidis P, Yaghmai V, Miller FH. Imaging of the urachus: anomalies, complications, and mimics. Radiographics 2016;36(7):2049–2063

Yu JS, Kim KW, Lee HJ, Lee YJ, Yoon CS, Kim MJ. Urachal remnant diseases: spectrum of CT and US findings. Radiographics 2001;21(2):451–461

■ Case 50

Castellino SM, Martinez-Borges AR, McLean TW. Pediatric genitourinary tumors. Curr Opin Oncol 2009;21(3): 278–283

Kobi M, Khatri G, Edelman M, Hines J. Sarcoma botryoides: MRI findings in two patients. J Magn Reson Imaging 2009;29(3):708–712

Parikh JH, Barton DPJ, Ind TEJ, Sohaib SA. MR imaging features of vaginal malignancies. Radiographics 2008;28(1):49–63, quiz 322

Van Rijn RR, Wilde JCH, Bras J, Oldenburger F, McHugh KM, Merks JH. Imaging findings in noncraniofacial childhood rhabdomyosarcoma. Pediatr Radiol 2008;38(6):617–634

■ Case 51

Kucera JN, Coley I, O'Hara S, Kosnik EJ, Coley BD. The simple sacral dimple: diagnostic yield of ultrasound in neonates. Pediatr Radiol 2015;45(2):211–216

Ladino Torres MF, DiPietro MA. Spine ultrasound imaging in the newborn. Semin Ultrasound CT MR 2014;35(6):652–661

Lowe LH, Johanek AJ, Moore CW. Sonography of the neonatal spine: part 1. Normal anatomy, imaging pitfalls, and variations that may simulate disorders. AJR Am J Roentgenol 2007;188(3):733–738

Rufener SL, Ibrahim M, Raybaud CA, Parmar HA. Congenital spine and spinal cord malformations—pictorial review. AJR Am J Roentgenol 2010;194(3, Suppl)S26–S37

Unsinn KM, Geley T, Freund MC, Gassner I. US of the spinal cord in newborns: spectrum of normal findings, variants, congenital anomalies, and acquired diseases. Radiographics 2000;20(4):923–938

■ Case 52

Aspelund G, Langer JC. Current management of hypertrophic pyloric stenosis. Semin Pediatr Surg 2007;16(1):27–33

Hernanz-Schulman M. Infantile hypertrophic pyloric stenosis. Radiology 2003;227(2):319–331

■ Case 53

Korkmaz AA, Yildiz CE, Onan B, Guden M, Cetin G, Babaoglu K. Scimitar syndrome: a complex form of anomalous pulmonary venous return. J Card Surg 2011;26(5):529–534

Vida VL, Padalino MA, Boccuzzo G, et al. Scimitar syndrome: a European Congenital Heart Surgeons Association (ECHSA) multicentric study. Circulation 2010;122(12):1159–1166

■ Case 54

Bousvaros A, Antonioli DA, Colletti RB, et al; North American Society for Pediatric Gastroenterology, Hepatology, and Nutrition; Colitis Foundation of America. Differentiating ulcerative colitis from Crohn disease in children and young adults: report of a working group of the North American Society for Pediatric Gastroenterology, Hepatology, and Nutrition and the Crohn's and Colitis Foundation of America. J Pediatr Gastroenterol Nutr 2007;44(5):653–674

Duigenan S, Gee MS. Imaging of pediatric patients with inflammatory bowel disease. AJR Am J Roentgenol 2012;199(4):907–915

Roggeveen MJ, Tismenetsky M, Shapiro R. Best cases from the AFIP: ulcerative colitis. Radiographics 2006;26(3):947–951

■ Case 55

Abramson SJ, Price AP. Imaging of pediatric lymphomas. Radiol Clin North Am 2008;46(2):313–338, ix

Gun F, Erginel B, Unüvar A, Kebudi R, Salman T, Celik A. Mediastinal masses in children: experience with 120 cases. Pediatr Hematol Oncol 2012;29(2):141–147

Ranganath SH, Lee EY, Restrepo R, Eisenberg RL. Mediastinal masses in children. AJR Am J Roentgenol 2012;198(3):W197–W216

■ Case 56

Dillman JR, Ladino-Torres MF, Adler J, et al. Comparison of MR enterography and histopathology in the evaluation of pediatric Crohn disease. Pediatr Radiol 2011;41(12):1552–1558

Furukawa A, Saotome T, Yamasaki M, et al. Cross-sectional imaging in Crohn disease. Radiographics 2004;24(3):689–702

Toma P, Granata C, Magnano G, Barabino A. CT and MRI of paediatric Crohn disease. Pediatr Radiol 2007;37(11):1083–1092

■ Case 57

Bendeddouche I, Jean-Luc BB, Poiraudeau S, Nys A. Anterior superior iliac spine avulsion in a young soccer player. Ann Phys Rehabil Med 2010;53(9):584–590

Naylor JA, Goffar SL, Chugg J. Avulsion fracture of the anterior superior iliac spine. J Orthop Sports Phys Ther 2013;43(3):195

■ Case 58

Lange R, Vogt M, Hörer J, et al. Long-term results of repair of anomalous origin of the left coronary artery from the pulmonary artery. Ann Thorac Surg 2007;83(4):1463–1471

Peña E, Nguyen ET, Merchant N, Dennie C. ALCAPA syndrome: not just a pediatric disease. Radiographics 2009;29(2):553–565

■ Case 59

Burton EC, Olson M, Rooper L. Defects in laterality with emphasis on heterotaxy syndromes with asplenia and polysplenia: an autopsy case series at a single institution. Pediatr Dev Pathol 2014;17(4):250–264

Pockett CR, Dicken B, Rebeyka IM, Ross DB, Ryerson LM. Heterotaxy syndrome: is a prophylactic Ladd procedure necessary in asymptomatic patients? Pediatr Cardiol 2013;34(1):59–63

■ Case 60

Chavhan GB, Parra DA, Oudjhane K, Miller SF, Babyn PS, Pippi Salle FL. Imaging of ambiguous genitalia: classification and diagnostic approach. Radiographics 2008;28(7):1891–1904

Stranzinger E, Strouse PJ. Ultrasound of the pediatric female pelvis. Semin Ultrasound CT MR 2008;29(2):98–113

Teixeira SR, Elias PC, Andrade MT, Melo AF, Elias Junior J. The role of imaging in congenital adrenal hyperplasia. Arq Bras Endocrinol Metabol 2014;58(7):701–708

■ Case 61

d'Almeida M, Jose J, Oneto J, Restrepo R. Bowel wall thickening in children: CT findings. Radiographics 2008;28(3):727–746

Kirkpatrick IDC, Greenberg HM. Gastrointestinal complications in the neutropenic patient: characterization and differentiation with abdominal CT. Radiology 2003;226(3):668–674

Thoeni RF, Cello JP. CT imaging of colitis. Radiology 2006;240(3):623–638

■ Case 62

Berrocal T, Lamas M, Gutiérrez J, Torres I, Prieto C, del Hoyo ML. Congenital anomalies of the small intestine, colon, and rectum. Radiographics 1999;19(5):1219–1236

Dalla Vecchia LK, Grosfeld JL, West KW, Rescorla FJ, Scherer LR, Engum SA. Intestinal atresia and stenosis: a 25-year experience with 277 cases. Arch Surg 1998;133(5):490–496, discussion 496–497

■ Case 63

Ozkoc G, Gonc U, Kayaalp A, Teker K, Peker TT. Displaced
supracondylar humeral fractures in children: open
reduction vs. closed reduction and pinning. Arch Orthop
Trauma Surg 2004;124(8):547–551

Simanovsky N, Lamdan R, Mosheiff R, Simanovsky N.
Underreduced supracondylar fracture of the humerus
in children: clinical significance at skeletal maturity.
J Pediatr Orthop 2007;27(7):733–738

■ Case 64

Bloom DC, Perkins JA, Manning SC. Management of
lymphatic malformations. Curr Opin Otolaryngol
Head Neck Surg 2004;12(6):500–504

Richter GT, Friedman AB. Hemangiomas and vascular
malformations: current theory and management.
Intern J Pediatr 2012:1–10

■ Case 65

Gipson MG, Cummings KW, Hurth KM. Bronchial atresia.
Radiographics 2009;29(5):1531–1535

Odev K, Guler I, Altinok T, Pekcan S, Batur A, Ozbiner H. Cystic
and cavitary lung lesions in children: radiologic findings
with pathologic correlation. J Clin Imaging Sci 2013;3:60

Rahalkar AM, Rahalkar MD, Rahalkar MA. Pictorial essay:
all about bronchial atresia. Indian J Radiol Imaging
2005;15(3):389–393

■ Case 66

Klein MJ, Siegal GP. Osteosarcoma: anatomic and histologic
variants. Am J Clin Pathol 2006;125(4):555–581

Murphey MD, Jelinek JS, Temple HT, Flemming DJ,
Gannon FH. Imaging of periosteal osteosarcoma:
radiologic-pathologic comparison. Radiology
2004;233(1):129–138

■ Case 67

Attenhofer Jost CH, Connolly HM, Dearani JA, Edwards
WD, Danielson GK. Ebstein's anomaly. Circulation
2007;115(2):277–285

Ferguson EC, Krishnamurthy R, Oldham SAA.
Classic imaging signs of congenital cardiovascular
abnormalities. Radiographics 2007;27(5):1323–1334

■ Case 68

De Mattos CB, Angsanuntsukh C, Arkader A, Dormans JP.
Chondroblastoma and chondromyxoid fibroma. J Am
Acad Orthop Surg 2013;21(4):225–233

Lehner B, Witte D, Weiss S. Clinical and radiological
long-term results after operative treatment of
chondroblastoma. Arch Orthop Trauma Surg
2011;131(1):45–52

■ Case 69

Bader RS, Chitayat D, Kelly E, et al. Fetal rhabdomyoma:
prenatal diagnosis, clinical outcome, and incidence
of associated tuberous sclerosis complex. J Pediatr
2003;143(5):620–624

Grebenc ML, Rosado de Christenson ML, Burke AP,
Green CE, Galvin JR. Primary cardiac and pericardial
neoplasms: radiologic-pathologic correlation.
Radiographics 2000;20(4):1073–1103,
quiz 1110–1111, 1112

■ Case 70

Aso C, Enríquez G, Fité M, et al. Gray-scale and color
Doppler sonography of scrotal disorders in children:
an update. Radiographics 2005;25(5):1197–1214

Coursey Moreno C, Small WC, Camacho JC, et al. Testicular
tumors: what radiologists need to know—differential
diagnosis, staging, and management. Radiographics
2015;35(2):400–415

Loberant N, Bhatt S, Messing E, Dogra VS. Bilateral
testicular epidermoid cysts. J Clin Imaging Sci 2011;1:4

Ross JH, Kay R. Prepubertal testis tumors. Rev Urol
2004;6(1):11–18

Sung EK, Setty BN, Castro-Aragon I. Sonography of the
pediatric scrotum: emphasis on the Ts—torsion, trauma,
and tumors. AJR Am J Roentgenol 2012;198(5):996–1003

■ Case 71

Stoker DJ. Osteopetrosis. Semin Musculoskelet Radiol
2002;6(4):299–305

Tolar J, Teitelbaum SL, Orchard PJ. Osteopetrosis. N Engl J
Med 2004;351(27):2839–2849

Case 72

Ebert EC. Gastrointestinal manifestations of Henoch-Schonlein purpura. Dig Dis Sci 2008;53(8):2011–2019

Peru H, Soylemezoglu O, Bakkaloglu SA, et al. Henoch-Schonlein purpura in childhood: clinical analysis of 254 cases over a 3-year period. Clin Rheumatol 2008;27(9):1087–1092

Case 73

de Lorijn F, Kremer LCM, Reitsma JB, Benninga MA. Diagnostic tests in Hirschsprung disease: a systematic review. J Pediatr Gastroenterol Nutr 2006;42(5):496–505

de Lorijn F, Reitsma JB, Voskuijl WP, et al. Diagnosis of Hirschsprung's disease: a prospective, comparative accuracy study of common tests. J Pediatr 2005;146(6):787–792

Case 74

Cloutier DR, Baird TB, Gormley P, McCarten KM, Bussey JG, Luks FI. Pediatric splenic injuries with a contrast blush: successful nonoperative management without angiography and embolization. J Pediatr Surg 2004;39(6):969–971

Holmes JF, Sokolove PE, Brant WE, et al. Identification of children with intra-abdominal injuries after blunt trauma. Ann Emerg Med 2002;39(5):500–509

Wegner S, Colletti JE, Van Wie D. Pediatric blunt abdominal trauma. Pediatr Clin North Am 2006;53(2):243–256

Case 75

Elhassanien AF, Alghaiaty HA. Joubert syndrome: clinical and radiological characteristics of nine patients. Ann Indian Acad Neurol 2013;16(2):239–244

McGraw P. The molar tooth sign. Radiology 2003;229(3):671–672

Poretti A, Huisman TAGM, Scheer I, Boltshauser E. Joubert syndrome and related disorders: spectrum of neuroimaging findings in 75 patients. AJNR Am J Neuroradiol 2011;32(8):1459–1463

Case 76

Fike FB, Mortellaro V, Juang D, St Peter SD, Andrews WS, Snyder CL. Neutropenic colitis in children. J Surg Res 2011;170(1):73–76

Kirkpatrick IDC, Greenberg HM. Gastrointestinal complications in the neutropenic patient: characterization and differentiation with abdominal CT. Radiology 2003;226(3):668–674

Mullassery D, Bader A, Battersby AJ, et al. Diagnosis, incidence, and outcomes of suspected typhlitis in oncology patients—experience in a tertiary pediatric surgical center in the United Kingdom. J Pediatr Surg 2009;44(2):381–385

Case 77

Berrocal T, Madrid C, Novo S, Gutiérrez J, Arjonilla A, Gómez-León N. Congenital anomalies of the tracheobronchial tree, lung, and mediastinum: embryology, radiology, and pathology. Radiographics 2004;24(1):e17

Konkin DE, O'hali WA, Webber EM, Blair GK. Outcomes in esophageal atresia and tracheoesophageal fistula. J Pediatr Surg 2003;38(12):1726–1729

Laffan EE, Daneman A, Ein SH, Kerrigan D, Manson DE. Tracheoesophageal fistula without esophageal atresia: are pull-back tube esophagograms needed for diagnosis? Pediatr Radiol 2006;36(11):1141–1147

Case 78

Brown ML, Burkhart HM, Connolly HM, et al. Coarctation of the aorta: lifelong surveillance is mandatory following surgical repair. J Am Coll Cardiol 2013;62(11):1020–1025

Tanous D, Benson LN, Horlick EM. Coarctation of the aorta: evaluation and management. Curr Opin Cardiol 2009;24(6):509–515

Case 79

Halaas GW. Management of foreign bodies in the skin. Am Fam Physician 2007;76(5):683–688

Horton LK, Jacobson JA, Powell A, Fessell DP, Hayes CW. Sonography and radiography of soft-tissue foreign bodies. AJR Am J Roentgenol 2001;176(5):1155–1159

Case 80

Akın MA, Akın L, Özbek S, et al. Fetal-neonatal ovarian cysts—their monitoring and management: retrospective evaluation of 20 cases and review of the literature. J Clin Res Pediatr Endocrinol 2010;2(1):28–33

Trinh TW, Kennedy AM. Fetal ovarian cysts: review of imaging spectrum, differential diagnosis, management, and outcome. Radiographics 2015;35(2):621–635

■ Case 81

Daneman A, Navarro O. Intussusception. Part 1: a review of diagnostic approaches. Pediatr Radiol 2003;33(2):79–85

Daneman A, Navarro O. Intussusception. Part 2: an update on the evolution of management. Pediatr Radiol 2004;34(2):97–108, quiz 187

Hryhorczuk AL, Strouse PJ. Validation of US as a first-line diagnostic test for assessment of pediatric ileocolic intussusception. Pediatr Radiol 2009;39(10):1075–1079

■ Case 82

Chung EM, Lattin GE Jr, Cube R, et al. From the archives of the AFIP: pediatric liver masses: radiologic-pathologic correlation. Part 2. Malignant tumors. Radiographics 2011;31(2):483–507

Roebuck DJ, Olsen Ø, Pariente D. Radiological staging in children with hepatoblastoma. Pediatr Radiol 2006;36(3):176–182

Roebuck DJ, Perilongo G. Hepatoblastoma: an oncological review. Pediatr Radiol 2006;36(3):183–186

■ Case 83

Kemp AM, Butler A, Morris S, et al. Which radiological investigations should be performed to identify fractures in suspected child abuse? Clin Radiol 2006;61(9):723–736

Offiah A, van Rijn RR, Perez-Rossello JM, Kleinman PK. Skeletal imaging of child abuse (non-accidental injury). Pediatr Radiol 2009;39(5):461–470

■ Case 84

Badger SA, Barclay R, Campbell P, Mole DJ, Diamond T. Management of liver trauma. World J Surg 2009;33(12): 2522–2537

Holmes JF, Sokolove PE, Brant WE, et al. Identification of children with intra-abdominal injuries after blunt trauma. Ann Emerg Med 2002;39(5):500–509

Yoon W, Jeong YY, Kim JK, et al. CT in blunt liver trauma. Radiographics 2005;25(1):87–104

■ Case 85

Berrocal T, López-Pereira P, Arjonilla A, Gutiérrez J. Anomalies of the distal ureter, bladder, and urethra in children: embryologic, radiologic, and pathologic features. Radiographics 2002;22(5):1139–1164

Das narla L, Doherty RD, Hingsbergen EA, et al. Pediatric case of the day. Prune-belly syndrome (Eagle-Barrett syndrome, triad syndrome). Radiographics 1998;18(5):1318–1322

Levin TL, Han B, Little BP. Congenital anomalies of the male urethra. Pediatr Radiol 2007;37(9):851–862, quiz 945

■ Case 86

Arora R, Trehan V, Kumar A, Kalra GS, Nigam M. Transcatheter closure of congenital ventricular septal defects: experience with various devices. J Interv Cardiol 2003;16(1):83–91

Minette MS, Sahn DJ. Ventricular septal defects. Circulation 2006;114(20):2190–2197

Penny DJ, Vick GW III. Ventricular septal defect. Lancet 2011;377(9771):1103–1112

■ Case 87

Epelman M, Daneman A, Navarro OM, et al. Necrotizing enterocolitis: review of state-of-the-art imaging findings with pathologic correlation. Radiographics 2007;27(2):285–305

Hsueh W, Caplan MS, Qu X-W, Tan XD, De Plaen IG, Gonzalez-Crussi F. Neonatal necrotizing enterocolitis: clinical considerations and pathogenetic concepts. Pediatr Dev Pathol 2003;6(1):6–23

Neu J, Walker WA. Necrotizing enterocolitis. N Engl J Med 2011;364(3):255–264

■ Case 88

Berrocal T, Torres I, Gutiérrez J, Prieto C, del Hoyo ML, Lamas M. Congenital anomalies of the upper gastrointestinal tract. Radiographics 1999;19(4):855–872

Choudhry MS, Rahman N, Boyd P, Lakhoo K. Duodenal atresia: associated anomalies, prenatal diagnosis and outcome. Pediatr Surg Int 2009;25(8):727–730

Escobar MA, Ladd AP, Grosfeld JL, et al. Duodenal atresia and stenosis: long-term follow-up over 30 years. J Pediatr Surg 2004;39(6):867–871, discussion 867–871

■ Case 89

Kleinman PK, Perez-Rossello JM, Newton AW, Feldman HA, Kleinman PL. Prevalence of the classic metaphyseal lesion in infants at low versus high risk for abuse. AJR Am J Roentgenol 2011;197(4):1005–1008

Thackeray JD, Wannemacher J, Adler BH, Lindberg DM. The classic metaphyseal lesion and traumatic injury. Pediatr Radiol 2016;46(8):1128–1133

■ Case 90

Han TI, Kim MJ, Yoon HK, Chung JY, Choeh K. Rhabdoid tumour of the kidney: imaging findings. Pediatr Radiol 2001;31(4):233–237

Lowe LH, Isuani BH, Heller RM, et al. Pediatric renal masses: Wilms tumor and beyond. Radiographics 2000;20(6):1585–1603

Winger DI, Buyuk A, Bohrer S, et al. Radiology-Pathology Conference: rhabdoid tumor of the kidney. Clin Imaging 2006;30(2):132–136

■ Case 91

Azouz EM, Saigal G, Rodriguez MM, Podda A. Langerhans' cell histiocytosis: pathology, imaging and treatment of skeletal involvement. Pediatr Radiol 2005;35(2):103–115

Hoover KB, Rosenthal DI, Mankin H. Langerhans cell histiocytosis. Skeletal Radiol 2007;36(2):95–104

■ Case 92

Carlyle BE, Borowitz DS, Glick PL. A review of pathophysiology and management of fetuses and neonates with meconium ileus for the pediatric surgeon. J Pediatr Surg 2012;47(4):772–781

Kao SCS, Franken EA Jr. Nonoperative treatment of simple meconium ileus: a survey of the Society for Pediatric Radiology. Pediatr Radiol 1995;25(2):97–100

■ Case 93

Cheng G, Soboleski D, Daneman A, Poenaru D, Hurlbut D. Sonographic pitfalls in the diagnosis of enteric duplication cysts. AJR Am J Roentgenol 2005;184(2):521–525

Onur MR, Bakal U, Kocakoc E, Tartar T, Kazez A. Cystic abdominal masses in children: a pictorial essay. Clin Imaging 2013;37(1):18–27

Ranganath SH, Lee EY, Eisenberg RL. Focal cystic abdominal masses in pediatric patients. AJR Am J Roentgenol 2012;199(1):W1–W16

■ Case 94

Chung EM, Cube R, Lewis RB, Conran RM. From the archives of the AFIP: pediatric liver masses: radiologic-pathologic correlation part 1. Benign tumors. Radiographics 2010;30(3):801–826

Kassarjian A, Zurakowski D, Dubois J, Paltiel HJ, Fishman SJ, Burrows PE. Infantile hepatic hemangiomas: clinical and imaging findings and their correlation with therapy. AJR Am J Roentgenol 2004;182(3):785–795

Roos JE, Pfiffner R, Stallmach T, Stuckmann G, Marincek B, Willi U. Infantile hemangioendothelioma. Radiographics 2003;23(6):1649–1655

■ Case 95

Meuwly JY, Lepori D, Theumann N, et al. Multimodality imaging evaluation of the pediatric neck: techniques and spectrum of findings. Radiographics 2005;25(4):931–948

Mittal MK, Malik A, Sureka B, Thukral BB. Cystic masses of neck: A pictorial review. Indian J Radiol Imaging 2012;22(4):334–343

■ Case 96

Beck BR, Bergman AG, Miner M, et al. Tibial stress injury: relationship of radiographic, nuclear medicine bone scanning, MR imaging, and CT Severity grades to clinical severity and time to healing. Radiology 2012;263(3):811–818

Gaeta M, Minutoli F, Scribano E, et al. CT and MR imaging findings in athletes with early tibial stress injuries: comparison with bone scintigraphy findings and emphasis on cortical abnormalities. Radiology 2005;235(2):553–561

■ Case 97

Dillman JR, Yarram SG, Hernandez RJ. Imaging of pulmonary venous developmental anomalies. AJR Am J Roentgenol 2009;192(5):1272–1285

Somerville J, Grech V. The chest x-ray in congenital heart disease 1. Total anomalous pulmonary venous drainage and coarctation of the aorta. Images Paediatr Cardiol 2009;11(1):7–9

■ Case 98

Krishnamoorthi R, Ramarajan N, Wang NE, et al. Effectiveness of a staged US and CT protocol for the diagnosis of pediatric appendicitis: reducing radiation exposure in the age of ALARA. Radiology 2011;259(1):231–239

Russell WS, Schuh AM, Hill JG, et al. Clinical practice guidelines for pediatric appendicitis evaluation can decrease computed tomography utilization while maintaining diagnostic accuracy. Pediatr Emerg Care 2013;29(5):568–573

Strouse PJ. Pediatric appendicitis: an argument for US. Radiology 2010;255(1):8–13

■ Case 99

Brofman N, Atri M, Hanson JM, Grinblat L, Chughtai T, Brenneman F. Evaluation of bowel and mesenteric blunt trauma with multidetector CT. Radiographics 2006;26(4):1119–1131

Butela ST, Federle MP, Chang PJ, et al. Performance of CT in detection of bowel injury. AJR Am J Roentgenol 2001;176(1):129–135

■ Case 100

Biyyam DR, Chapman T, Ferguson MR, Deutsch G, Dighe MK. Congenital lung abnormalities: embryologic features, prenatal diagnosis, and postnatal radiologic-pathologic correlation. Radiographics 2010;30(6): 1721–1738

Daltro P, Werner H, Gasparetto TD, et al. Congenital chest malformations: a multimodality approach with emphasis on fetal MR imaging. Radiographics 2010;30(2):385–395

Index

Locators refer to case number. Locators in boldface indicate primary diagnosis.